# THE ULTIMATE SIRTFOOD DIET 2021 EDITION

*TO ACTIVATE YOUR SKINNY GENE, BURN, FAT, LOSE WEIGHT, PREVENT DISEASES AND IMPROVE YOUR LIFE. INCLUDING 30 DAYS MEAL AND 30 EASY AND HEALTHY RECIPES*

GUENDA MOSS

# The Ultimate

# Sirtfood Diet

## 2021 Edition

Including 30 Days
Meal and
30 Easy and Healthy
Recipes

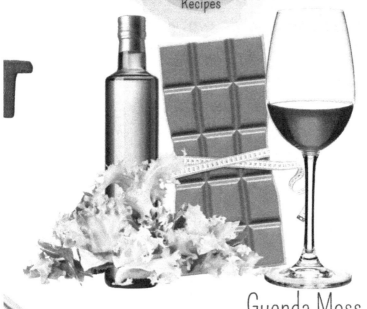

Guenda Moss

# THE ULTIMATE SIRTFOOD DIET 2021 EDITION

*To Activate Your Skinny Gene, Burn, Fat, Lose Weight, Prevent Diseases And Improve Your Life. Including 30 Days Meal and 30 Easy and Healthy Recipes*

GUENDA MOSS

liable for any hardship or damages that may befall them after undertaking information described herein.

Additionally, the information in the following pages is intended only for informational purposes and should thus be thought of as universal. As befitting its nature, it is presented without assurance regarding its prolonged validity or interim quality. Trademarks that are mentioned are done without written consent and can in no way be considered an endorsement from the trademark holder.

# INTRODUCTION

When we cut back on calories, it makes a lack of vitality that enacts what is known as the "skinny quality." This triggers a heap of positive changes. It places the body into a kind of endurance mode where it quits putting away fat and typical development forms are required to be postponed. Rather, the body directs its concentration toward consuming its stores of fat and turning on ground-breaking housekeeping qualities that fix and revive our cells, successfully giving them a spring cleaning. The consequence is weight loss and improved protection from infection.

Sirtfoods are a newfound group of miracle foods. Sirtfoods are especially wealthy in uncommon supplements that, when we devour them, can initiate a similar skinny qualities in our bodies that calorie limitation does. These qualities are known as sirtuins. They originally became exposed in a milestone concentrate in 2003 when analysts found that resveratrol, a compound found in red grape skin and red wine, significantly expanded the life expectancy of yeast.2 Incredibly, resveratrol had a similar impact on life span as calorie limitation, yet this was accomplished without reducing vitality intake. From that point forward studies have demonstrated that resveratrol can expand life in worms, flies, fish, and even honeybees.3 And from mice to people, early-stage studies show resveratrol secures against the antagonistic impacts of fatty, high-fat, and high-sugar consumes fewer calories; advances sound maturing by deferring age-related sicknesses; and increments fitness.4 fundamentally it has been appeared to impersonate the impacts of calorie limitation and exercise.

With its rich resveratrol content, red wine was hailed as the first Sirtfood, clarifying the medical advantages connected to its utilization, and even why individuals who drink red wine gain less weight.5 However, this is just the start of the Sirtfood story.

Launched initially in 2016, the Sirtfood diet stays a hotly debated issue and includes followers embracing a diet rich in 'Sirt foods'. As indicated by the diet organizers, these unique nourishments work by initiating explicit proteins in the body called sirtuins. Sirtuins are accepted to shield cells in the body from dying when they are under pressure and are thought to control irritation, digestion, and the maturing procedure. It's the idea that sirtuins impact the body's capacity to consume fat and lift digestion, bringing about a seven-pound weight loss seven days while looking after muscle. However, a few specialists accept this is probably not going to be exclusively fat loss, yet will rather reflect changes in glycogen stores from skeletal muscle and the liver.

With the discovery of resveratrol, the universe of health research was on the cusp of something significant, and the pharmaceutical business wasted no time committing. Specialists started screening a huge number of various chemicals for their capacity to activate our sirtuin qualities.

This uncovered various common plant mixes, not only resveratrol, with noteworthy sirtuin-initiating properties. It was likewise found that a given food could contain an entire range of these plant mixes, which could work in show to both guide assimilation and amplify that food's sirtuin-enacting effect. This had been one of the large riddles around resveratrol. The researchers exploring different avenues regarding resveratrol frequently expected to use far higher portions than we know give an advantage when devoured as a feature of red wine. However, just as resveratrol, red wine contains a variety of other normal plant mixes, including high measures of piceatannol just as quercetin, myricetin, and epicatechin, every one of which was appeared to freely actuate our sirtuin qualities and, increasingly significant, to work in coordination.

The issue for the pharmaceutical business is that they can't advertise a group of supplements or foods as the following big blockbuster drug. So all things considered they contributed a huge number of dollars to create and lead trials of manufactured mixes with expectations of revealing a Shangri-la pill. At this moment different studies of sirtuin-enacting drugs are in progress for a large number of constant sicknesses, just as the first-historically speaking FDA-endorsed trial to research whether a medication can slow maturing.

As enticing as that may appear, if history has shown us anything, it's that we ought not to hold out a lot of trust in this pharmaceutical ambrosia. Over and over the pharmaceutical and health enterprises have attempted to imitate the advantages of foods and diets through isolated medications and supplements. Furthermore, over and over its missed the mark. Why sit tight ten or more years for the authorizing of these purported wonder drugs, and the unavoidable symptoms they bring, when right now we have all the inconceivable advantages accessible readily available through the food we eat?

So while the pharmaceutical business tirelessly seeks after a drug like a magic bullet, we need to retrain our attention on diet. For simultaneously those efforts were in progress, the scene of nourishing exploration was additionally shifting, bringing up some enormous issues of its own. Red wine to the other side, were there different foods with significant levels of these extraordinary supplements fit for enacting our sirtuin qualities? Also, assuming this is the case, what were their consequences for activating fat loss and battling sickness?

Dietitian Emer Delaney says:

'From the start, this isn't a diet I would prompt for my customers. Expecting to have 1000kcal for three back to back days is very troublesome and I accept most of the individuals would be not able to accomplish it. Taking a look at the list of nourishments, you can see they are the kind of things that

---

13

regularly show up on a 'healthy food list'; anyway it is smarter to empower these as a major aspect of a healthy adjusted diet. Having a glass of red wine or a modest quantity of chocolate every so often won't do us any mischief - I wouldn't suggest them regularly. We ought to likewise be eating a blend of various fruits and vegetables not only those on the list.

'As far as weight loss and boosting digestion, individuals may have encountered a seven-pound weight loss on the scales, yet I would say this will be liquid. Burning and losing fat requires significant investment so it is very improbable this weight loss is lost fat. I would be extremely careful of any diet that suggests quick and abrupt weight loss as this just isn't attainable and will more than likely be lost of fluid. When individuals come back to their standard eating patterns, they will recover the weight. Gradual weight loss is the key and for this we have to limit calories and increment our movement levels. Eating balanced standard meals comprised of low GI nourishments, lean protein, fruit and vegetables, and keeping all-around hydrated is the most secure approach to get thinner.'

This diet depends on research about sirtuins (SIRTs), a group of seven proteins found in the body that has been appeared to manage a variety of capacities, including digestion, irritation, and lifespan.

Certain normal plant mixes might have the option to expand the degree of these proteins in the body, and nourishments containing them have been named "Sirt foods."

# Chapter 1: SIRTFOOD

Sirtfoods are recently found group of nutrient-rich foods which appear to be able to 'actuate' the body's skinny genes (otherwise called sirtuins), similarly as fasting diets do, with a similar scope of advantages, however without the regular drawbacks of fasting diets, for example, irritability, hunger, and muscle loss.

By eating a diet rich in Sirtfoods, it is asserted that participants will get thinner, gain muscle, look and feel good and possibly live a longer and increasingly healthy life.

### WHAT IS SIRTFOOD DIET?

The Sirtfood Diet is the better approach to move weight rapidly without radical dieting by initiating the same 'skinny gene' pathways generally just induced by fasting and exercise. Certain foods contain synthetic compounds called polyphenols that put mild stress on our phones, turning on genes that copy the impacts of exercise and fasting. Foods rich in polyphenols-including dark chocolate, kale, and red wine-trigger the sirtuin pathways that effect digestion, mood and aging. A diet rich in these sirtfoods launches weight reduction without sacrificing muscle while maintaining ideal health.

Add healthy sirtfoods to your diet for successful and sustained weight reduction, incredible vitality and sparkling health. Switch on your body's fat-burning powers, supercharge weight reduction and help stave off disease with this simple-to-follow diet created by the specialists in nutritional prescription who proved the effect of Sirt foods. Dark chocolate, kale, coffee - these are foods that actuate sirtuins and switch on the alleged 'skinny gene' pathways in the body. The Sirtfood Diet gives you a straightforward, healthy way for eating for weight reduction, delicious simple-to-make plans and an maintain plan for delayed success. The Sirtfood Diet is a diet of incorporation not avoidance, and sirtfoods are widely affordable and available. This is a diet that urges you to get your fork and knife, and appreciate eating delicious healthy food while seeing the wellbeing and weight reduction benefits.

## HEALTH BENEFITS OF SIRT FOOD DIETS

In our Sirtfood Diet trial members lost an amazing 7 pounds over the underlying 7 days remembering increments for muscle and muscle work. This emotional impact on fat-consuming, while advancing muscle, is one reason that our Sirtfood-based diet has gotten so well-known with anybody needing to get lean and fit as a fiddle, much the same as the tip-top competitors and models who have supported along these lines of eating. Alongside fat consumption, Sirtfoods likewise have the one of a kind capacity to normally satisfy hunger making them the ideal answer for accomplishing a solid weight and continuing it long term.

However, to consider it absolutely as a weight loss diet is to overlook the main issue. This is a diet that has a lot to do with health as waistlines. Expanded energy, more clear skin, feeling progressively alert, and better rest are the charming 'symptoms' from thusly of eating. In some cases the advantages are considerably increasingly striking, remembering situations where following the diet for the more extended term has turned around metabolic sicknesses. Such is the health-enhancing impacts that reviews demonstrate them to be all the more remarkable then professionally prescribed medications in preventing chronic illness, with benefits in diabetes, coronary illness and Alzheimer's to give some examples. It's no big surprise that it is entrenched that the way of life eating the most Sirtfoods has been the least leanest and healthiest in the world.

The main concern is clear: If you need to accomplish a more energetic, slender, and more beneficial body, and establish the systems for long-lasting health and protection from infection, at that point the Sirtfood Diet is for you.

### WHAT ARE THE ADVANTAGES?

You will get in shape if you follow this diet intently. "Whether or not you're eating 1,000 calories of tacos, or 1,000 calories of snickerdoodles, 1,000 calories of kale, you will shed pounds at 1,000 calories!" says Dr. Youdark

The advantages of Sirtfood likewise incorporate the accompanying;

- Drive your weight loss from fat and not muscle
- Ensure you look better, feel much improved and have more vitality
- Prepare your body for long term weight loss achievement
- Stop you encountering extreme fasting or intense appetite
- Free you from depleting exercise meetings
- Be a springboard for a more drawn out, more advantageous and infection-free life

## WHY SIRTFOOD OVER ANY OTHER DIET?

Sirtfoods are a recently found group of regular plant foods, known as sirtuin activators, which switch on our 'skinny' qualities – similar qualities enacted by fasting and exercise.

Unlike other diet plans, which are explicitly outfitted towards unhealthy and dramatic weight loss, the Sirtfood Diet is great if you essentially need to boost your resistant system, pack in certain nutrients and feel somewhat healthier.

Alongside this fat-burning impact, sirtfoods additionally have the unique capacity to ¬naturally control hunger and increase muscle function – making them the ideal answer for accomplishing a healthy weight.

Undoubtedly, their health-boosting impacts are incredible to such an extent that a few studies have shown them to be more powerful than professionally prescribed medications in forestalling constant infection, with apparent ¬benefits in diabetes, coronary illness and ¬Alzheimer's disease.

No big surprise cultures eating the most sirtfoods – including Italy and Japan – are the least fatty and most healthy on the planet. What's more, that is the reason we've formulated a diet based around them.

# CHAPTER 2: HEALTHY SIRT FOODS

While it may not be a diet that is beneficial to follow exactly, there are a lot of valid justifications to include a significant number of the center Sirtfoods in a weight loss plan, including kale, berries, green tea, ginger, turmeric and olive oil.

Here's an introduction on a portion of the top Sirtfoods — simply make certain to appreciate them with regards to a fair diet with a variety of other healthy nourishments.

1. Chia Seeds

In the realm of Sirtfoods, chia seeds are noted to be a moderate sirtuin-enacting food that the authors of The Sirtfood Diet depict in their book as what might be compared to going for a stroll as opposed to getting in an extraordinary sweat session at the gym.

There's no healthy proof to help this claim, however, there's no discussion that chia seeds pack a huge amount of nourishment into a little bundle, making them an effective method to stack up on key supplements like fiber (around 10 grams for every ounce) and folate (around 14 micrograms), per the USDA. Chia is additionally a decent source of plant protein. Simply sprinkle the seeds over a smoothie bowl, add to smoothies or blend into oats.

## 2. Cinnamon

In an investigation published in April 2017 in Biochemistry and Molecular Biology, analysts utilized a PC model to check whether cinnamon actuated sirtuins and discovered promising associations. This doesn't demonstrate anything yet, however, it's a fascinating structure obstruct for future research.

However, cinnamon despite everything makes the Sirtfoods list since it offers incredible polyphenols, which are plant compounds with antioxidant and anti-inflammatory properties. What's more, some exploration seems to propose that cinnamon can assist control with blood sugar by easing back carb absorption and improving how the body reacts to insulin, as indicated by the Mayo Clinic.

Cinnamon goes extraordinary in espresso, hot cocoa, collard greens, broiled squash, soups, smoothies, and flavor rubs for lean pork.

## 3. Cocoa

The proposed sirtuin-actuating supplement in cocoa is epicatechin, an incredible sort of antioxidant additionally found in tea and grapes.

As a polyphenol-rich food, cocoa may help advance healthy bloodstream, per an April 2017 Cochrane audit — not that you required another motivation to appreciate chocolate. Simply recall that the advantages are from the cocoa plant, not all the additional sugar, salt, and fat in handled pieces of candy.

Search for the most noteworthy rate dark chocolate you can discover to receive the most rewards.

## 4. Olive Oil

The alleged sirtuin-enacting polyphenols in additional virgin olive oil are oleuropein and hydroxytyrosol. What we can be sure of is that olive oil is a key part of the heart-healthy Mediterranean diet, which can likewise bolster a weight-the board plan.

It's additionally wealthy in monounsaturated fats, which can help improve cholesterol levels, particularly when they supplant immersed fat or refined carbs, per the American Heart Association.

## 5. Berries

Berries, for example, strawberries, raspberries, and blackberries are rich in polyphenols, so it does not shock anyone that berries are antioxidant whizzes, per the Mayo Clinic. They're likewise rich in fiber and vitamin C.

New berries are great all alone, and healthy berries can be advantageously delighted in all year in a group satisfying smoothie or a suddenly new salsa.

## 6. Kale

A cup of kale has twofold the day's nutrient A, and more nutrient C than an orange, per the USDA.

To prepare kale, remove stems, fold, and cut across into strips (chiffonade) before kneading for a couple of moments with your preferred dressing. Include these marinated kale strips and whatever fruits you have around with your preferred grain, for example, sorghum, farro, wheat berry, or freekeh, for a brisk and healthy entire grain serving of salad.

## 7. Red Wine

Red wine made its name in health circles for containing the polyphenol resveratrol. Observational research in people proposes that moderate intake could have medical advantages for heart health and possibly for life span and brain health, as well, as indicated by Harvard Health Publishing.

As a conventional piece of the Mediterranean diet, it's intended to be delighted in with food in fitting sums (e.g., one 5-ounce glass for ladies every day). It's not directly for everybody, and there are numerous different approaches to eat and drink for good health for any individual who wants to swear off wine in any way, shape, or form.

## THE TOP 20 SIRTFOODS

Lots of nourishments contain sirtuin-enacting supplements, yet some contain more than others. In their book 'The Sirtfood Diet', the writers of the diet list the 20 best Sirtfoods, these are: birds eye chilies, buckwheat, escapades, celery, cocoa, espresso, additional virgin olive oil, green tea, kale, lovage,

Medjool dates, parsley, red chicory, red wine, rocket, soy, strawberries, turmeric and pecans.

The Sirtfood Diet was made by nutritionists Aiden Goggins and Glen Matten. They were so intrigued by the capability of Sirtfoods, they made a diet based around expanding Sirtfood consumption and gentle calorie limitation. They at that point tried this diet on members from an elite London rec center and were stunned by their discoveries. Gym members lost a normal of 7lbs in the initial 7 days, despite not expanding their degrees of activity. Not exclusively did the members lose a generous measure of weight, yet they additionally picked up muscle (ordinarily the inverse happens when abstaining from excessive food intake) and announced critical upgrades in by and large health.

The diet is part of 2 stages. Stage 1: the 7 day 'hyper success stage', which joins a Sirtfood-rich diet with moderate calorie limitation, and Phase 2: the 14-day' maintenance stage', where you merge your weight loss without confining calories.

Stage 1 OF THE SIRT FOOD DIET

During the initial 3 days, calorie intake is confined to 1,000 calories (along these lines, still more than on a 5:2 fasting day). The diet comprises of 3 Sirtfood-rich green juices and 1 Sirtfood-rich feast and 2 squares of dark chocolate.

During the remaining 4 days, calorie intake is expanded to 1,500 calories, and every day the diet involves 2 Sirtfood-rich green juices and 2 Sirtfood-rich suppers.

During stage 1 you are not permitted to drink any liquor, yet you can drink water, tea, coffee, and green tea freely.

Stage 2 OF THE SIRT FOOD DIET

Stage 2 doesn't concentrate on calorie limitation. Every day includes 3 Sirtfood-rich meals and 1 green juice, in addition to the alternative of 1 or 2 Sirtfood nibble snacks, whenever required.

In stage 2 you are permitted to drink red wine, however with some restraint (the suggestion is 2-3 glasses of red wine every week), just as water, tea, espresso, and green tea.

## IS THERE AN EATING PLAN FOR THE SIRT FOOD DIET?

Truly, there is a useful graph mentioning to you what you can eat every day and when. The book has all the plans you will require for the initial three weeks. There is a meat/fish alternative and a veggie lover/vegetarian choice for consistently. Practically all the plans are without gluten and there are sans dairy choices consistently meaning this is a diet that will work for the vast majority.

## WHAT HAPPENS AFTER YOU HAVE FINISHED THE SIRT FOOD DIET?

The Sirtfood Diet isn't intended to be a one-off 'diet' but instead a lifestyle. You are empowered, when you've finished the initial 3 weeks, to keep eating a diet rich in Sirtfoods and to keep drinking your every day green juice. There are even a few plans for Sirtfood pastries! The creators of The Sirtfood Diet recommend that Phases 1 and 2 can be repeated as and when important for a health support, or if things have gone somewhat off course.

## DOES THE SIRT FOOD DIET WORK?

All things considered, it does as per their numerous superstar supports. The subsequent book has supported by David Haye (Heavyweight Boxer), Lorraine Pascale (TV Chef and Food Writer), Jodie Kidd (Model), Sir Ben Ainslie (Olympic Gold Medallist) and an entire pile of different big names who all case that the Sirtfood Diet has helped them get in shape, manufacture muscle and look and feel great. Although my preferred support is certainly the one which is ascribed to a spouse of a member and which peruses 'Bless your heart! My significant other is looking extra hot.'

Anyway there is a touch of me which is somewhat suspicious – possibly the diet works for a celebrity who has coordinated diet instructing and no uncertainty a fitness coach as well. In any case, will the Sirtfood Diet work for a conventional individual like me? All things considered, there is just a single method to address that question. I have concluded that for the following 3 weeks I will follow Phase 1 and 2 of the Sirtfood Diet and report back on how it goes.

I will keep all of you refreshed on Twitter, Facebook, or Instagram about how I am jumping on every day and afterward compose a week after week roundup every week on a Monday morning to share how my week has gone. I would adore for you to tail me/support me/and for the most part collaborate with me on my excursion.

Or then again why not go along with me? The Sirtfood Diet book is generally accessible and contains all you have to think about the diet. Furthermore, on the off chance that you need more formula motivation there is The Sirtfood Diet Recipe Book too which contains bunches of additional plans just as more counsel and tips.

### SIRT FOOD GREEN JUICE RECIPE

The Sirtfood-rich green juice is a significant piece of the Sirtfood-diet, so I figured it is useful to include the formula here. Regardless of whether you have no goal of following the diet, the juice is stuffed loaded with supplements and would be an incredible expansion to a customary diet. One significant thing to note: I have examined cautiously and you completely need to make this in a juicer, NOT a blender (or a Nutribullet or food processor or whatever else other than a juicer). I have given the two different ways out and can report that the mixed rendition is frightful tasting sludge; the squeezed adaptation is a sensibly good tasting juice!

# Chapter 3: THE SKINNY GENE

The ALK (anaplastic lymphoma kinase) quality is the variation that encourages protection from weight gain, regardless of what diet an individual has. It diminishes individuals stay thin, possibly opening another frontier in medicines for weight.

The gene assumes a role in resisting weight gain in the metabolically healthy, slight individuals. It is found in the nerve center, the area in the brain answerable for controlling hunger and how an individual controls fat.

The ALK quality makes a protein called anaplastic lymphoma kinase, which is associated with cell growth. The quality is likewise connected to specific diseases and distinguished as a driver of tumor growth.

## ALK VARIATIONS

The group broke down the DNA of more than 47,000 individuals between the ages of 20 and 44 years of age. They took a look at the data from Estonia's biobank, an organic database gathered from a huge level of the Estonian population.

The analysts recognized thin, healthy people in the most minimal sixth percentile of weight. The benchmark group, then again, were those in the 30th and 50th percentile. Individuals from the 95th percentile were labeled as the obese group. The group distinguished the variations of qualities that seemed to happen all the more frequently in the thin group.

In the wake of examining the database, the group found that a few variations in the ALK quality were attached to low defenselessness to weight gain in normally dainty individuals. The group likewise found that erasing the quality had prompted more slender flies. Further, mice hereditarily changed to do not have the ALK quality additionally demonstrated stamped protection from weight.

## THERAPEUTICS TARGETING THE GENE

The group says that therapeutics focusing on the gene may assist researchers with handling and battle stoutness later on. If there could be an approach to close down the ALK quality or lessen its capacity, at any rate, individuals can remain thin. At present, ALK medicines, for example, inhibitors are being utilized in cancer.

Further research is expected to check whether tranquilize inhibitors are successful for this reason before they are trialed in people. The group anticipates the second phase of the study, which means to compare the discoveries and biobank records on the health, DNA, and movement levels of different populaces over the globe.

The group additionally plans to concentrate on how neurons that express the ALK direct the mind at an atomic level to adjust metabolism and advance thinness.

The advancement came when we found that the advantages of fasting were interceded by activating our ancient sirtuin qualities, otherwise called the "skinny gene". At the point when energy is hard to find, precisely as found in calorie limitation, an expanded measure of pressure is put on our cells. This is detected by the sirtuins, which at that point get turned on and communicate amazing signs that fundamentally adjust how our cells act.

Sirtuins ramp up metabolism, increment the effectiveness of muscles, switch on fat consumption, lessen inflammation and fix any harm in cells. As a result, sirtuins make us fitter, less fatty and more beneficial.

ARE THE SKINNY GENE A THING

Throughout the years, different research trials have been directed to help decide whether there are extremely 'skinny genes. For what reason do a few people truly battle with their weight though others appear to eat what they need without gaining any additional weight? While diet and way of life are the undeniable contributing components, weight differences in animals have given us the motivation to accept there might be more to it than that; and maybe there's likewise a greater amount of an inward driving variable - genes.

Throughout the years, up to 50 different genes have been discovered which are without a doubt thought to have an impact on our weight and body piece. Huge numbers of these are expected to impact how we ingest and use fats, and even have an impact on our appetite.

One of the latest revelations was the 'skinny gene' which has been alleged 'adipose'1. This was initially found in natural fruit flies, yet has additionally been found in rodents and people. If the quality is turned on, the individual is bound to be 'skinny', while if it's turned off, we're bound to store progressively fat, or fat tissue. In any case, strangely the 'skinny gene' isn't believed to be just turned on or off, however it might be turned on to fluctuating degrees in various people.

## THE ROLE OF GUT BACTERIA

Just as inalienable genes having an impact on our body weight, there are possibly other inside impacts as well, for example, the balance of bacteria in our gut.

Gut bacteria preliminaries have demonstrated that the pervasiveness of particular kinds of microbes is connected to various body loads among people2, and although it's not surely known how precisely these functions, we realize that these microorganisms can discharge synthetic chemicals which can conceivably adjust our genes too.

Although gut microorganisms can be affected from birth (with cesarean conceived babies found to have an alternate equalization from those conceived normally), there are a lot of steps you can take as far as your diet and way of life to help advance a healthier balance of gut bacteria and, accordingly, possibly impact your weight thusly as well – another significant thought!


### THE INFLUENCE OF DIET

Although individuals are getting increasingly intrigued by genetics and what genes we may or not have –you're left with your genetic makeup. In any case, what I truly need to pressure is that you can impact these genes in various manners:

1 - The power of nourishment could turn genes on or off

We realize that diet and our condition can impact our genes straightforwardly. Strikingly the 'skinny gene' is believed to be turned on to various degrees in various individuals – so everybody has it, we simply need to impact it.

2 - Genetic components aren't the most important thing in the world

Although certain individuals might be pre-arranged to specific things because of their genes, with regards to bodyweight (and loads of different factors, for example, disease states), there are heaps of motivation to accept that we can defeat even genes, because of outside impacts, for example, diet and way of life, at any rate to a limited degree! For by far most individuals, dealing with their diet or taking a shot at more exercise will have the desired impact when done perfectly.

3 - Genes alone aren't to be faulted for the ongoing increment in weight

Just accusing our genes risks being somewhat of a cop-out with regards to body weight. As both corpulence and the related illnesses, for example, diabetes has expanded exponentially in all pieces of the world over a similar time frame in recent years, we realize that genes aren't the entire story. This pattern proposes diet, dietary patterns and social impacts are substantially more liable to assume the primary job.

Are there explicit diets that can impact our 'skinny genes'?
There is by all accounts a consistent flow of new craze diets accessible these days and it very well may be hard to tell which, if any of them, are probably going to be appropriate for supporting your health or explicit weight reduction goals.
Regarding conceivably impacting that ' skinny gene' the Sirtfood Diet has been given some uncommon consideration as of late. The Sirtfood Diet is alleged because it is wealthy in nourishments high in exceptional chemical compound called sirtuin activators. Sirtuins are a particular class of compounds which are thought to have useful impacts in the body and the nourishments they can be found in incorporate bunches of healthy things, for example, green tea, dull chocolate, citrus natural products, apples, turmeric, blueberries, kale, and red wine.
Presently, although I'm supportive of remembering these nourishments for your diet, it must be stated, the exploration

is somewhat crude regarding the particular impacts that these food sources can have, because of their sirtuin activator content. The Sirtfood Diet rules are commonly truly controlled, genuinely severe with no place for breathing space, they include cutting calories drastically and substituting appropriate dinners for juices. Although these sorts of plans can now and again be useful in the present moment for instance, as a feature of a delicate detox, longer-term it's probably not going to be so maintainable. It's significantly more reasonable to embrace a way of life which underpins your health and body weight in the long term.

SUMMARIZING AND MAKING A MOVE

In this way, in case you're frantic to make a move and bolster a more beneficial you, skinny genes or not, here's my recommendation:

1 – Incorporate the Sirtfood diet parts into your diet at any rate
Instead of following an overly severe system and prescriptive recipes, why not simply put forth an attempt to incorporate a greater amount of the components of the Sirtfood diet in your system at any rate? Regardless of whether the sirtuins are having explicit activities in the body, these nourishments are stuffed brimming with nutrients, minerals, and antioxidants

which are significant for supporting healthy substantial procedures and a buzzing metabolism.

I truly accept that cooking from new is the way into a healthy body weight. It's all the prepared nourishments with concealed sugars, salts, fat (and the rest!) that are considerably more liable to add to us heaping on the pounds. Eat new, start arranging and preparing your dinners and you'll before long feel and notice the distinction.

2 – Don't disregard the solid fats

Something that the Sirtfood diet is ostensibly missing is a decent portion of healthy fats. Individuals are frequently prone to avoid fats, particularly when attempting to shed pounds, yet in all honesty, we need healthy fats to help our digestion and remain lean!

An ongoing report likewise featured this idea and found that older individuals who effectively presented an extra 300 calories for each day from walnuts had no negative impacts on body weight or body piece which incorporates fat dispersion. This is truly encouraging, and simply think about the potential outcomes if you incorporated these and cut out something less accommodating! So no reason, get consolidating those fats!

3 – Regardless of your qualities, assume responsibility for your way of life

Indeed, even the specialists have concurred that there's nothing you can't do to impact your genes. So regardless of whether we are inclined to certain body types or disease states, it just methods we are at more danger of these various states, it isn't unavoidable that we'll get influenced. Subsequently, our diet, every day propensities, and way of life variables would all be able to have an impact and even little changes might have the universe of effect.

One top tip to consider is how much water you drink. We realize that water impacts each arrangement of our body, and research has recommended that this basic constituent of our diet could be urgent for supporting our qualities and by and large health.

Not exclusively are the advantages of water there, however, if you drink more water you're more averse to drink different things – other conceivably progressively harmful things. There's been a consistent increment in the utilization of calorific beverages as of late, and with calories come all the sugar, fake sugars, caffeine, and liquor which are normal segments of beverages that aren't water – all of which aren't probably going to help your digestion! In this way, drink up, and include a cut of lemon or some other organic product in case you're battling at first

4 – Herbal partners

In case you're attempting to get in shape, although there's not prone to be any handy solution as far as products (yes individuals, diet and way of life truly is critical!) there are a couple of zones you could focus on to help your advancement:

Support your metabolism with Kelp

Supporting your thyroid organ and digestion is consistently a significant thought in case you're chipping away at your weight. Particularly in the way to deal with menopause, or if your hormones have been playing up as of late, your thyroid may require some delicate help and our Kelp tablets with a reasonable portion of iodine can be an invite expansion!

## BOLSTER YOUR STOMACH WITH UNPLEASANT HERBS

Supporting your stomach with some severe herbs, for example, Yarrow guarantees that you are retaining all the basic supplements from your food and benefiting as much as possible from them. Magnesium helps bolster insulin affectability and B nutrients help us to change over our food into energy– these are only two supplements worth referencing which are excessively significant for supporting a healthy body weight.

## BOLSTER YOUR GUT WITH PREBIOTICS

All together for the bacteria in your gut to endure and carry out their responsibility adequately (metabolism is a major piece of this), they should be in an appropriate domain. Including a decent portion of L+ lactic corrosive to you day by day system by utilizing Molkosan can help make only that, and you'll unquestionably need to do this first before considering presenting any probiotics supplements.

The change to Sirtfoods

"Sirtfoods" are the notable methods for enacting our sirtuin genes in the most ideal manner. These are the marvel nourishments especially rich in explicit regular plant chemicals, called polyphenols, which can address our sirtuin genes, turning them on. They emulate the impacts of fasting and practice and in doing so bring amazing advantages by helping the body to all the more likely control glucose levels, consume fat, form muscle, and lift health and memory.

Since they're fixed, plants have built up an exceptionally advanced stress-reaction system and produce polyphenols to assist them with adjusting to the difficulties of their condition. At the point when we devour these plants, we likewise expend these polyphenol supplements. Their impact is significant: they enact our natural pressure reaction pathways.

While all plants have pressure reaction frameworks, just certain ones have created to deliver essential measures of sirtuin-actuating polyphenols. These plants are Sirt foods.

---

Their revelation implies that rather than severe diets or burdensome exercise programs, there's currently a progressive better approach to actuate your sirtuin qualities: eating a diet inexhaustible in Sirt foods. The best part is that this one includes putting (Sirt)foods onto your plate, not taking them off.

# Chapter 4: HOW TO FIGHT AGAINST OBESITY

1. Focus on the nutritional content of your food

Lack of nutritious diet can cause obesity. You can reduce your calorie intake by making healthier choices and eating a balanced diet, and reduce the threat of obesity.

Make sure you have plenty of fruits and vegetables in your shopping cart, so you can conveniently catch a piece of fruit or vegetable if hunger hits. You will target at having five different pieces of fruit and vegetables every day.

Scan the food and beverage labels and find out exactly what's in them, so you can make educated choices when you purchase them.

Be mindful of the calories you consume. You don't have to be on a diet but knowing how many calories you eat will help you eat no more than your body needs.

Eat smaller meals daily to avoid hunger because this helps keep your metabolism up without snacking foods with a high sugar content. Don't feel the urge to finish everything on your plate if you start feeling full.

Swap junk foods, processed foods, and takeaways for healthier substitutes. Don't store at home unhealthy choices.

Do healthier choices when eating out. Numerous cafés now detail their meals' calories and dietary substance and that will assist you with settling on an informed choice.

2. Avoid unhealthy and sugar laden drinks

Numerous delicate and alcoholic drinks have a high sugar content. An excess of sugar can prompt weight gain and obesity. In a split second powered beverages, squashes, juice drinks, and fizzy drinks that contain a great deal of added sugar however not many supplements. Natural fruit juices and smoothies are frequently thought to be a solid option but they contain sugar so you ought to confine your admission to a joined aggregate of 150ml per day.

You will strive to drink about 6 to 8 glasses of fluid a day. Water is best, it's a healthy, inexpensive choice to quench your thirst. It does not have any calories, but sugars. Other healthier options include lower fat milk and sugar-free beverages including coffee and tea.

Alcohol calories are 'vacuum calories,' they have no nutritional value. Your body can't store alcohol so processes like nutrient absorption and burning fat are interrupted to get rid of the alcohol. You can still drink alcohol but you are aiming for less drink. Many alcoholic brands now have 'light' or low alcohol alternatives that can be tried or chosen for a low-calorie mixer like a diet coke. Drinking water in alcoholic drinks will cut down on the amount of units you consume.

3. Learn about and understand your eating habits

Research on obesity has found that obese people can suffer from many emotional problems regarding their weight and body image.

Conversing with an expert about your eating pattern can regularly assist you with understanding them more and with this information you can find a way to beat gorging or eating solace. You can need to converse with a family member or friend and get from them the assist you with expecting to make them feel better.

4. Obesity treatment

If you are obese and have attempted to lose weight by diet and exercise, but have not reached or sustained a successful weight loss level, or you have a severe health problem that might be changed if you lose weight, such as type 2 diabetes or high blood pressure, then weight loss treatment or surgery may be the best choice for you.

HOW TO BEAT OBESITY

Williamsburg, Va. — Experts agree: obesity in our nation has become an almost epidemic crisis. So at a ground-breaking obesity conference earlier this month, academic, health care, business, media and policy leaders gathered to discuss solutions to the issue.

---

The concept behind the Time / ABC News Conference on Obesity was to look from both angles at the problems. The aim was to encourage the participants to return and make a difference to their communities.

So, what's the latest tactic in the obesity war? Here are a few accentuations:

Taking a Village — NOW!

In every talk, "Time is of the essence" was a message repeated as was the call for prevention — beginning with our children. Experts accepted that our children would be the original to die sooner than their parents due to the adult-like diseases that go along with obesity in their childhood.

There's always been consensus that working together is the best way to win the fight on obesity. If we are going to make a difference, the food industry, government, health care providers, students, neighborhoods and parents all need to join hands.

If we don't, we'll all pay dearly, both with our money and health. The economic drain caused by health issues associated with obesity is devastating. Today, we can barely bear the prices, let alone the estimated 10 years from now.

What's On the Menu?

Are carbohydrates, protein or fats making us fat? The bottom line is that you will gain weight if you eat too much of any or all of those nutrients. There's nothing special about low-carb diets, the glycemic index, or too much protein. Calories are what counts, and fad diets function (at least in the short term) as they minimize the overall quantity of calories you consume, easy and clear.

The most convincing presentations at the summit advocated a diet high in complex carbohydrates, healthy fats, lean protein, and plenty of fruits and vegetables and discouraged processed carbs, sugars, trans fats, and saturated fats — just as we do at the WebMD Weight Loss Clinic.

No matter what else you consume, there's no such thing as a balanced diet without a big dose of produce — where you'll find over 1,000 health-promoting, disease-protective substances (antioxidants, phytochemicals, isoflavones, etc.), says Dean Ornish, MD.


THE BLAME GAME

You could predict a decent amount of finger-pointing and allegations at a meeting with so many dietary heavy-hitters in attendance. But most agree that "the blame game" is a waste of energy and time.

Obesity is a complicated issue, and not the responsibility of any party, food, company or advertisement. We need to help people take responsibility for what they eat instead of blaming each other, and inspire them to get some exercise.

James O. Hill, PhD, Americaonthemove.org's co-founder, wants us all to put on pedometers and walk, walk, walk, add extra steps to our everyday lives in whatever way we can.

Consolidate 10,000 stages for each day with a healthy diet, and you will be well on your way toward losing weight and improving your health.


## ONE SIZE DOES NOT FIT ALL

Of this, the message is that there is no solution to the issue. Each of us needs to find the healthy eating plan that fits best for our lifestyles and build more healthy behaviors — like daily physical activity.

It will contain lots of complex carbohydrates, fruits , vegetables, healthy fats and lean protein, no matter which diet we adopt. And the amount of processed carbohydrates, trans-fats and saturated fats should be reduced.

Progress depends on how ready each of us is to commit to a healthier lifespan. We've discovered that weight management isn't just about education; most of us know that a healthy diet and daily exercise are the road to better health. Now, we just need to do this — and get our friends, family and neighbors to join us in fighting obesity.


## SIRTUINS AND MUSCLE FAT

In the body, there is a family of genes that function as guardians of our muscle and when under stress avoid its breakdown: the sirtuins. SIRT1 is a strong Muscle Breakdown Inhibitor. So long so SIRT1 is triggered, the muscle breakdown is prevented even when we are fasting and we start burning fat for fuel.But SIRT1 's benefits aren't done with maintaining muscle mass. Sirtuins actually work to improve our skeletal muscle mass. We need to delve into the fascinating world of stem cells to understand how that process works. Our muscle contains a special form of stem cell which is called a satellite cell that regulates its growth and regeneration.

Most of the time, satellite cells only sit there quietly but they are stimulated when the muscle gets weakened or stressed. Via things like weight training this is how our muscles get bigger. SIRT1 is important for activating satellite cells, and muscles are substantially weaker without their operation since they no longer have the capacity to properly grow or regenerate. However, we are giving a boost to our satellite cells by increasing SIRT1 activity which encourages muscle growth and recovery.

### SIRTFOODS VS FASTING

This leads us to a big question: if sirtuin activation increases muscle mass, then why do we lose muscle when we fast? After all, fasting activates our sirtuin genes as well. And herein lies one of the massive drawbacks of fasting.

This leads to a big question: if activation of the sirtuin increases muscle mass, why do we lose muscle when we fast?

Fasting also stimulates our sirtuin genes, after all. And therein lies one of fasting 's big drawbacks.

Bear with us as we dig through the workings of this. Not all skeletal muscles are created equal to each other. We have two key forms, called type-1 and type-2 conveniently. Type-1 muscle is used for movements of longer length, while the type-2 muscle is used for brief bursts of more vigorous activity. And here's where it gets intriguing: fasting increases SIRT1 activity only in type-1 muscle fibers, not type-2. But type-1 muscle fiber size is preserved and even significantly increases when we fast.8 Unfortunately, in complete contrast to what happens in type-1 fibers during fasting, SIRT1 decreases rapidly in type-2 fibres. It means that fat burning slows down, and muscle breaks down to provide heat, instead.

But fasting for the muscles is a double-edged sword, with our type-2 fibers taking a hit. Type-2 fibers form the bulk of our concept of muscle. And even though our type-1 fiber mass is growing, with fasting we also see a substantial overall loss of muscle. If we were able to avoid the breakdown, it would not only make us look aesthetically good but also help to encourage more loss of weight. And the way to do this is to combat the decrease in SIRT1 in muscle fiber type-2 that is caused by fasting.

Researchers at Harvard Medical School tested this in an elegant mice study and found that the signals for muscle breakdown were turned off and no muscle loss occurred by stimulating SIRT1 activity in type-2 fibers during fasting.

The researchers then went a step further and tested the effects of increased SIRT1 activity on the muscle when the mice were fed rather than fasted, and found it stimulated very rapid growth of the muscle. In a week, muscle fibers with elevated levels of SIRT1 activity displayed an impressive weight gain of 20 per cent.

Such results are very close to the outcome of our Sirtfood Diet trial, but in turn, our research has been milder. After increasing SIRT1 activity after consuming a diet rich in syrtfoods, most participants had no muscle loss — and for others, it was only a moderate strong, muscle mass that actually increased.

# Chapter 5: THE SIRT DIET PRINCIPLES

With a normal 650 million powerful adults globally, it's basic to find shrewd counting calories and exercise systems that are possible, don't prevent you from claiming all that you acknowledge, and don't anticipate that you should rehearse all week. The Sirtfood diet does just that. The idea is that certain nourishments will dynamic the 'slim quality' pathways which are regularly incited by fasting and exercise. Luckily certain nutrition and drink, including dark chocolate and red wine, contain engineered substances called polyphenols that order the characteristics that duplicate the effects of movement and fasting.

### EXERCISE DURING THE UNDERLYING SCARCELY ANY WEEKS

During the primary week or two of the diet where your calorie admission is reduced, it is sensible to stop or reduce practice while your body adjusts to less calories. Check out your body and if you feel depleted or have less imperativeness than anticipated, don't work out. Or maybe ensure that you remain focused on the guidelines that apply to a strong way of life, for instance, including palatable step by step levels of fiber, protein, and results of the soil.

## WHEN THE DIET TRANSFORMS INTO A WAY OF LIFE

At the point when you do practice it's basic to eat up protein ideally an hour after your exercise. Protein fixes muscles after exercise, reduces irritation, and can support recovery. There is a collection of recipes that fuse protein which will be perfect for post-practice usage, for instance, the Sirt stew con Carne or the turmeric chicken and kale serving of salad. If you need something lighter you could endeavor the Sirt blueberry smoothie and include some protein powder for included bit of leeway. The sort of health you do will be down to you, anyway exercises at home will allow you to pick when to work out, the sorts of exercises that suit you and are short and accommodating.

The Sirtfood diet is an inconceivable way to deal with changing your dietary patterns, shed pounds, and feel increasingly beneficial. The hidden very few weeks may provoke you yet it's basic to check which nourishments are perfect to eat and which luscious recipes suit you. Be big-hearted to yourself in the underlying scarcely any weeks while your body adjusts and takes practice basic if you choose to do it in any way shape or form. If you are starting at now someone who conservatives or extraordinary exercise, at that point it may be that you can carry on as ordinary, or manage your health according to the alteration in diet. Thus similarly as with any diet and exercise changes, it's about the individual and how far you can drive yourself.

Minerals and supplements for which women may require supplements fuse calcium, iron, Vitamins B6, B12, and D. Men, in any case, need to concentrate on fiber, magnesium, Vitamins B9, C, and E.

That reason applies to weight loss eats less moreover. Individuals' nutrition necessities influence which weight loss counts calories are progressively convincing for each sex.

In case you're like by far most, you've seen a shocking number of weight-loss tasks and examples go to and fro; all of them have their advantages and all of them work — by chance. Weight the executives and therapeutic experts battle by and large that the profound established, demonstrated mix of good food and normal exercise is the best way to deal with sufficiently shed pounds and keep it off.

# Chapter 6: LOSE FAT AND NOT MUSCLE

## FAT LOSS VS WEIGHT LOSS: IT'S NOT THE SAME

People say they want to shed some pounds. The thing is, "weight" can be a few different things. For instance:

People frequently say they want to get in shape. This thing is, "weight" can be a couple of various things. For instance:

- Muscle.
- Fat.
- Glycogen.
- Poop.
- Water.

If all you care about is losing weight, you might get food poisoning and poop your brains out, or sit in a sauna and sweat a great deal. You could remove a leg and you'll lose "weight" fine and dandy. (Disclaimer: please do not do that)

However, If you are reading this, I will accept that you would prefer not to lose any of this other stuff. Or maybe, what you need to do here is lose fat, NOT muscle.

## HOW FAT LOSS HAPPENS

Loss of fat has only one significant necessity: a caloric shortage.

A caloric deficit or shortage is the state when you expend fewer calories than your body consumes for vitality.

When this occurs, it powers your body to locate an elective wellspring of vitality to consume for fuel rather, and that will principally wind up being your stored body fat.

How Muscle Loss Occurs

Ideally, the ONLY thing your body would burn while in a caloric shortage is your stored body fat.

In any case, it turns out there's a subsequent vitality source available: your muscle tissue.

And keeping in mind that you may need your body to just burn fat and not burn any muscle at all, actually, your body doesn't generally give a crap about what you desire.

All it thinks about is keeping you alive (fun actuality: your body can not tell if you're in a caloric shortage because you are trying to lose some fat, or because you are at risk of starving to death), and to get that going, it will need to take some stored energy/vitality from somewhere.

That can mean muscle, fat, or a mix of both.

How To Prevent It

What you have to do here is change your diet and exercise in ways that will cause your body more likely to burn body fat, and less likely to burn muscle fat.

How do you do this, you ask?

Here are the eight best ways to lose fat without losing muscle:

1. Eat A Sufficient Amount Of Protein

Your total daily protein consumption is the most significant dietary factor when it comes to maintaining muscle.

It's not specific food decisions, or when you eat, or how regularly you eat, or supplements, or carbs, or even the specific size of your caloric deficiency.

Healthfully, the greatest key to losing fat without losing muscle is eating an adequate amount of protein every day.

Even without a legitimate weight training routine, a greater amount of the weight you lose will be muscle mass because of a higher protein consumption.

Along these lines, the initial step to any muscle-preserving diet will eat a perfect measure of protein constantly.    How much is that precisely? Indeed, given the available research...

For most individuals, between the range of 0.8 – 1.3g of protein per pound of your present body weight is the sweet spot for preserving muscle during fat loss.

2. Increase or Maintain Strength Levels

Would you be amazed if I disclosed to you that utilizing a very much structured weight training program is essential for losing fat while maintaining muscle?

No? I didn't think so.

What may amaze you, however, is that it's more than simply "utilizing an exercise program" or "doing strength training" that gives the muscle-holding benefits we desire.

The primary training boost for building muscle is dynamic strain overload, which implies bit by bit getting more grounded over time.

For instance, if you lift some weights for the same number of reps for the following 20 years, your body will still have no reason to build extra muscle. However, if you gradually lift the same weight for more reps, or lift more weight, your body would then have more reason to build more muscle.

What's more, this same idea applies to keeping up muscle also. You will probably give your body a reason to maintain the muscle mass it already has.

How do you do that?

At least, aim to maintain your present strength levels all through the length of the weight loss program, or, if conceivable, increment them. Doing so gives a "muscle support" signal that tells your body it needs to maintain the muscle it has or build more.

Consider it like this. When your body is searching for an alternative fuel source to consume for vitality, and it can pick muscle mass or body fat for that reason, it will be more averse to pick muscle (and bound to pick fat) if it sees there is a reason behind keeping the muscle around.

3.  Try not to Reduce Calories By Too Much

As I clarified before, a caloric shortage should be available with the goal for you to lose body fat, and that implies you're going to need to diminish your calorie consumption to some degree.

The thing is, that level of shortage can be a wide range of various sizes going from pointlessly little to too much.

And keeping in mind that diverse deficit sizes can suit certain individuals in specific circumstances more so than others, research and certifiable experience fit toward a moderate deficiency being perfect for some, reasons, including preserving muscle.

Specifically...

The perfect caloric deficiency for the vast majority is between 15-25% beneath their maintenance level, with an even 20 percent regularly being a decent beginning stage.

In this way, for instance, if your upkeep level happened to be 2500 calories and you needed to make a 20 percent deficiency, you'd aim to eat around 2000 calories every day.

Why Not Use A Larger Deficit?

This is the moment that you might be asking why a bigger shortage isn't being utilized. All things considered, wouldn't diminish your calories by more than this make weight loss happen significantly quicker?

That is correct, it surely would.

However, remember this isn't just about "weight loss." Our objective is more explicit than that. We need to lose fat... and do it without losing muscle.

What's more, for that reason, enormous shortages, low-calorie diets, and "quick" weight loss will be bad ideas for many people.

Indeed, this kind of thing is an impractical notion for some reasons, as it can worsen:

- Hormonal adaptations.
- Hunger
- Mood
- Metabolic Slowdown
- Sleep Quality
- Water Retention
- Fatigue and Lethargy
- Recovery and Performance
- Reproductive Function and Libido
- Sustainability and Adherence
- Disordered Eating Habits

4.  Decrease Weight Training Frequency And/Or Frequency

A caloric shortage is a vitality shortage, and keeping in mind that this is awesome (and required) for losing any measure of body fat, it's not perfect for boosting weight training recuperation and performance.

This is something we just discussed a second prior as far as bigger deficits having a bigger negative effect in such manner.

However, even with only a moderate deficit set up, there is probably going to still be some drop-off in recuperation/performance contrasted with when you're at maintenance or in an overflow.

Why does this matter, you ask?

Since the exercise routine you were (or would be) utilizing with extraordinary accomplishment for an objective like building muscle under non-deficit conditions presently can be a lot for your body to deal with in the energy-deficient state it is in currently.

Also, that sort of situation? That is what makes strength to be lost. What's more, when strength is lost in a deficiency, muscle loss is what ordinarily follows.

If you're utilizing an exercise routine that includes more volume (reps, sets, and works out) or potentially recurrence (exercises every week) than you can handle, you may see things getting more difficult for you, or see that you're getting weaker, or that reps are diminishing, or that progress is relapsing, or that weight on the bar should be decreased, and in the end... that muscle is being lost.

How To Prevent It

How do you avoid all of this?

This could mean decreasing training volume (for example doing somewhat fewer sets), decreasing training volume (for example utilizing a 3-day exercise routine rather than a 5-day exercise routine), or a blend of both.

The specific changes you should make (or whether any modifications really should be made at this stage) relies upon the particular exercise routine you're utilizing and your recuperation capabilities.

5.   Get Pre And Post Workout Nutrition Right

Your pre and post-workout/exercise meals, otherwise known as the meals you eat before and after your session, are not exactly as very significant as the vast majority portray them.

They are only one of numerous components of your diet that are auxiliary to your all-out calorie and macronutrient consumption (for example fat, protein, and carbs), which is consistently what makes a difference most with regards to losing fat or maintaining/building muscle.

Having said that, your pre and post-workout meals matter still.

No, they are not capable of breaking or making your success, but they are capable of giving advantages that can improve your exhibition during an exercise, and upgrade recuperation related training adjustments after an exercise.

---

What's more, since we know that 1) recovery and performance are diminished to a certain level while we're in a deficiency, and 2) this can expand the danger of muscle loss... it's quite safe to state that these are benefits we need to get.

Anyway, what do you have to do to get them?

Expend a decent amount of carbs and protein within one to two hours before and after your workout/exercises.

6. Incorporate Calorie or Refeeds Cycling

As I've clarified all through this chapter, the basic act of being in a drawn-out caloric shortage or deficit makes an assortment of changes happen that expand the danger of muscle loss.

From hormonal adjustments, to expanded fatigue and lethargy, to a decrease in recuperation and performance... it all makes losing muscle-bound to occur.

Luckily for us, there are strategies we can use to help limit these impacts or possibly even reverse them.

These strategies include:
• Calorie Cycling
• Refeeds
• Diet Breaks

Refeeds and calorie cycling permit us to briefly stop our shortage by deliberately eating more calories – particularly from carbs, as carbs have the greatest positive effect on a hormone called leptin – to get back up to our maintenance level or into an excess.

In addition to being valuable from the angle of making your diet progressively sustainable, these strategies will likewise serve to recharge muscle glycogen stores (which assists with performance and strength) and positively affect various psychological and physiological factors that are contrarily affected during a shortage or deficit.

How To Do It

• Refeeds

Refeeds can be done a couple of various ways, however, it's a 24 hour time of being out of your shortage and eating somewhere close level and 500 calories above it (with the expansion in calories coming principally through carbs). I have discovered one refeed day per each week as a decent frequency for those with a normal measure of fat to lose, and once every other week is useful for those with an above-average amount to lose.

• Calorie Cycling

Calorie cycling is numerous refeed days (for instance 2-3) over seven days, often arranged so that you are taking more calories on your exercise days, and less calories on your rest days, with the particular daily amount balanced varying to still have the proposed total weekly net shortage/deficit at long last.

Along these lines, with an average weight loss diet, you would be devouring about the same amount of macronutrients and calories constantly, and be in a steady caloric shortage day after day.

Refeeds and calorie cycling change this by embeddings non-deficit days to help diminish the negative impacts a prolonged deficit can have, and make us bound to retain muscle while losing fat.

7. Take Diet Breaks When Needed

Take what we just talked about refeeds and calorie cycling, however, envision their positive advantages being more significant.

Imagine that as opposed to diminishing the negative impacts of a prolonged deficit, we could reverse those impacts to some level.

That is the full diet break.

A diet break is commonly a one to two-week time-frame where you come out of the deficit and back up to your maintenance level with the end goal of quickly permitting many of the things that suck about fat loss. (for example metabolic and hormonal adaptations) to recoup a piece and return to normal (or possibly, closer to normal).

This is advantageous for some reasons, one of which is forestalling muscle loss.

How To Do It

To take a diet break, increment your calorie consumption (essentially through extra carbs) with the goal that you are at your maintenance level each day for a time of one to two weeks.

Diet break frequency ought to be reliant on personal preferences/needs, and how much fat you need to lose. Generally, once every six to sixteen weeks tend to be perfect for most (maybe every 6-12 weeks if you have less to lose, and each ten to sixteen weeks if you have more to lose).

Much the same as with refeeds and calorie cycling, diet breaks are likewise a major piece of my Superior Fat Loss program.


8.   Avoid Excessive Amounts Of Cardio

Cardio is extra exercise... and extra exercise requires extra recuperation.

While this can be dangerous at any time and under any circumstance, we realize the potential is higher when we're in the energy insufficient (and recuperation-impaired) state we should be in for fat loss to happen. Which we are.

This implies, the more workout we do, the more danger we posture to our capacity to adequately recoup, both regarding the body parts being utilized the most (regularly the legs with most types of cardio), just as the central nervous system (CNS)... which influences everything.

Furthermore, if recuperation starts to suffer, performance and strength will suffer. What's more, when performance and strength suffer, so will your capacity to assemble or maintain muscle while losing fat.

Precisely how much of an effect cardio has in such manner is difficult to state, as it relies upon the specific duration, intensity, and frequency of the activity being finished.

For instance...

• Three cardio sessions every week will have less of an effect than five to seven sessions.

• Thirty minutes of cardio will have less of an effect than one hour to two hours.

• A low-intensity activity – like strolling – would have next to zero effect contrasted with a more moderate-intensity activity, for example, jogging.

• And neither would have nearly as quite a bit of an effect as something with a high intensity – like HIIT (high-intensity interval training, for example, running) – which can nearly be like adding weight training exercise as far as the pressure and stress it puts on your body and how recovery-intensive it is.


Farewell Fat, Hello Muscle!

There you have it... the best things you can do to guarantee you lose fat without losing muscle simultaneously.

While the initial two things (adequate protein consumption and keeping up/expanding strength) are the most significant, most logically bolstered, and generally beneficial in this regard, I've discovered that actualizing the entirety of the recommendations in this book is what produces the best outcomes.

# Chapter 7: PRINCIPLES OF HEALTHY WEIGHT LOSS AND FAT LOSS

With regards to losing weight and fat, the details do not make a difference. It's the principles that count.

"It's the people who understand the principles who do well long-term," says Arthur Agatston.

Each real nutritional professional, regardless of whether a well known diet master or an agent of the clinical nutritional establishment, concurs that there are some crucial standards of healthy weight loss that apply to everybody. Regardless of the amount they are camouflaged, these standards are at the center of every great diet plan, be it a dietician's arrangement or a bestseller's. Also, no one accomplishes perpetual weight loss and ideal health without complying with these standards, intentionally or unknowingly. While there appears to be no right approach to eat for heathy weight and fat loss, you should know about the fundamental principles. This will assist you with staying away from those diet plans that do in truth break them and pick the particular plan that is ideal for you.

"It's those that comprehend the principles who do well long haul," says Arthur Agatston.

1. Balance

Pundits of famous diets as often claim that such diets support lopsided eating by announcing certain nourishments and even whole food classes off-limit. The model they constantly point to is the notorious cabbage soup diet. In any case, that is an entirely extraordinary example.

What the pundits neglect is the fact that the average American diet is somewhat lopsided to begin with: heavy on fried foods, animal foods, processed foods, vegetables, whole grains, and sweet and light fruits. It's difficult to find a well-known diet that doesn't urge dieters to expend an assortment of new, natural plant food, and along these lines support, if not a totally balanced diet, then at least an increasingly balanced one.

In Cracking the Metabolic Code,a naturopathic physician and a pharmacist, known as  James LaValle, who is based in in Cincinnati, OH, clarifies how supplement imbalances of different sorts can prompt weight gain, and then again, how improving supplement balance can encourage weight loss.

To give one model, an underactive thyroid organ is a typical reason for moderate digestion and, subsequently, weight gain. Among the numerous components that can bring down thyroid capacity are elevated levels of adrenal pressure hormones, for example, cortisol, and as LaValle calls attention to, "Eating a great deal of sugar triggers the discharge of adrenal hormones." The average American diet contains 18 percent sugar. The average well-known diet assuredly doesn't!

2. Nutrient Timing

A spate of late research has indicated that when we eat is nearly as significant as what we eat regarding streamlining our body composition. "We've discovered that it's fundamental to coordinate vitality consumption with vitality use. "Calories are put to their most ideal use when they are devoured at times when there is a solid demand for them in the body." explains John Ivy, Ph.D. and coauthor of Nutrient Timing (Basic Health, 2004).

Morning is a period of moderately high caloric demand. Calories expended in the morning are almost certain than calories devoured later in the day to be utilized for vitality than put away as fat. Actually, a study from the University of Massachusetts found that the individuals who routinely skip breakfast are 4.5 times bound to be overweight than the individuals who eat it most mornings.

Eating smaller meals more often (five or six times each day) is another demonstrated method to all the more likely facilitate food admission with vitality needs. As indicated by statistical data, the average American eats three enormous meals every day.

3. Self-Monitoring

Research has indicated that focusing on what you eat is one of the more powerful approaches to diminish your caloric admission. Self-monitoring techniques are a key propensity among individuals from the National Weight Control Registry, an exploration pool comprising thousand people who have lost a normal of 66 pounds each and kept the weight off an average of six years. "They're exceptionally aware of their eating," says Suzanne Phelan, Ph.D., a representative for the NWCR. "About half of them report that they are as still counting fat grams and calories."

Another helpful self-monitoring propensity that is basic among both the NWCR subjects and those seeking after weight loss on famous diets is weighing. As indicated by Phelan, this propensity permits the subjects of her study to stay away from the guileful upward creep that is the undoing of numerous initial fruitful diets. "Since they are weighing themselves as regularly as they do, they can get these slips," she says. "In the event that they do something about it right away, they're substantially more prone to be fruitful in the long haul."

4.  Selective Restrictions

Every famous diet has a forbidden foods list. The particular food and food types that make the rundown and how severely they are forbidden differ from one program then onto the next. The Atkins diet forbids all high-sugar nourishments. The Ornish diet prohibits animal foods. Diminish D'Adamo's blood type diet disallows a long list of apparently irrelevant foods for every one of the four fundamental bloods types.

No weight loss diet can prevail without limitation of the foods that are generally responsible for making enormous body fat stores. Majority of standard nutrition professionals concur that the "bad fats" found in many animal foods and processed foods and the "bad carbs" in processed foods and desserts are the primary culprits. Strangely, about all the members of the NWCR decide to confine admission of high-fat foods. "Just 7% are on a low-carb diet," says Phelan.

Standard nutrition specialists caution against taking food limitations excessively far. "To dispose of specific food and food groups, particularly those that individuals enjoy, is a recipe for disaster and can prompt feelings of hardship, also wholesome awkward nature," says Elisa Zied, M.S., R.D., a representative for the American Dietetic Association.

James LaValle recommends soft limitations to his customers and in the numerous nitrition books he's composed. "You get masters who state, 'You can never eat another pastry again,'" he says. "That sets up a guilt complex in individuals." When the alternatives are all or nothing, there is no happy medium between being on the diet and unhappy and being off it totally.

5. Low Caloric Density

The idea of energy density or caloric density alludes to the quantity of calories per unit volume in a particular food. A food that has a great deal of calories in a smaall region is said to have high caloric density. Since water and dietary fiber are non-caloric, foods that contain a ton of water and additionally fiber will in general have low caloric density. Generally, processed foods are calorically dense, while leafy foods, with their high fiber and water content, are less dense.

Caloric density is significant for those looking to lose weight and fat because research has indicated that individuals will in general eat a reliable volume of food paying little heed to the quantity of calories it contains. In a Penn State study, ladies were fed either a low-density, medium-density, or high-density meal three times each day. The subjects in each of the three groups ate a similar load of food, however the ladies eating the high-density meal took in 30 percent a larger number of calories than the ladies eating the low-density meals.

## 6. Consistency

Eating healthy isn't like a vaccine: one shot and you're secured forever. Rather it requires an every day, long lasting commitment. There is developing proof that the more consistent you are in your eating habits, the more prominent your odds of maintaining a healthy body weight.

Once more, the members of the National Weight Control Registry set a model. "One of our latest discoveries is that they do keep up a consistent eating pattern," says Phelan. "In contrast to numerous dieters, they tend to eat the equivalent during the week as on the ends of the week. The same holds for these special seasons versus the rest of the year. They generally have a steady eating pattern constantly."

A constant myth of dieting is that the individuals who make long haul progress start off with a progressively moderate, gradual methodology than the crash dieters who take on extreme limitations just to bail out after several weeks or months and regain their weight. As indicated by Phelan, there is no proof that the long-term successes start off in an unexpected way. The genuine contrast is that they essentially continue doing what they started doing!

## 7. Motivation

Why are a few dieters able to keep up their healthy new lifestyle uncertainly while most others peter out following weeks or months? This is presently one of the hottest inquiry in weight reduction research. There is no definitive answer, however there are signs that it's generally about motivation.

Particular sorts of triggers for weight reduction diets are bound to yield long haul accomplishment than others. For instance, "One thing we've found is that individuals who have clinical triggers for their weight reduction are more successful in the long haul than individuals who don't," says Phelan. There's not at all like a brush with death to keep you on the narrow and straight path of healthy eating.

More proof for the motivation clarification originates from the fact that pretty much every other clarification can be eliminated.

It is regularly expected that successful dieters have progressively natural self discipline. However, most members of the NWCR really bombed in a few weight reduction activities before they finally succeeded, showing that something about their conditions as opposed to their mental make up was the key.

Bad genes that fight weight reduction are additionally habitually blamed. But, says Phelan, "A significant number of [the NWCR members] have parents who were overweight or were overweight themselves as kids, which recommends they may have a hereditary inclination to obesity, however they still manage to shed pounds."

# Chapter 8: 30 DAYS MEAL

**WEEK 1**

DAY 1

Breakfast: one serving Pineapple Green Smoothie (297 calories)

A.M. Snack: three to four cup raspberries (48 calories)

Lunch: 1 serving Tuna-Spinach Salad (375 calories)

P.M. Snack: 3/4 cup red wine (85 calories)

Dinner: one serving Dijon Salmon with Green Bean Pilaf (442 calories)

DAY 2

Breakfast: one serving Muffin-Tin Quiches with Smoked Cheddar and Potato (238 calories)

A.M. Snack: dark chocolate (230 calories)

Lunch: one serving Instant Pot White Chicken Chili Freezer Pack with a side of two celery stalks and three Tbsp. hummus (346 calories)

P.M. Snack: two plums (61 calories)

Dinner: onw serving Chicken and Vegetable Penne with Parsley-Walnut Pesto (514 calories)

DAY 3

Breakfast: one serving Muffin-Tin Quiches with Smoked Cheddar and Potato (238 calories)

A.M. Snack: 1 peach (68 calories)

Lunch: one serving Instant Pot White Chicken Chili Freezer Pack with a side of two celery stalks and three Tbsp. hummus (346 calories)

P.M. Snack: three cup blackberries and six walnut halves (125 calories)

Dinner: one serving Greek Turkey Burgers with Spinach, Feta & Tzatziki with a side of two cups mixed greens topped with one Tbsp. Basil Vinaigrette (442 calories)

DAY 4

Breakfast: one serving Muffin-Tin Quiches with Smoked Cheddar and Potato (238 calories)

A.M. Snack: red wine (85 calories)

Lunch: one serving Instant Pot White Chicken Chili Freezer Pack with a side of two celery stalks and three Tbsp. hummus (346 calories)

P.M. Snack: one square of dark chocolate (230 calories)

Dinner: one serving Meal-Prep Falafel Bowls with Tahini Sauce (500 calories)

DAY 5

Breakfast: one serving Pineapple Green Smoothie (297 calories)

A.M. Snack: two plums (61 calories)

Lunch: one serving Instant Pot White Chicken Chili Freezer Pack with a side of two celery stalks and three Tbsp. hummus (346 calories)

P.M. Snack: three to four cup red wine 85 calories)

Dinner:onw serving Vegetarian Spaghetti Squash Lasagna with a side of two cups mixed greens topped with onw Tbsp. Basil Vinaigrette (416 calories)

Meal-Prep Tip: Prepare onw serving of Creamy Blueberry-Pecan Overnight Oatmeal to have for breakfast tomorrow.


DAY 6

Breakfast: onw serving Creamy Blueberry-Pecan Overnight Oatmeal (291 calories)

A.M. Snack: three to four cup red wine (85 calories)

Lunch: 1 serving Tuna-Spinach Salad (375 calories)

P.M. Snack: 3/4 cup red wine (85 calories)

Dinner: one serving Hasselback Caprese Chicken with 1 1/2 cups Roasted Fresh Green Beans (443 calories)


DAY 7

Breakfast: one serving Pineapple Green Smoothie (297 calories)

A.M. Snack: dark chocolate (230 calories)

Lunch: one serving Tuna-Spinach Salad (375 calories)

P.M. Snack: one cup sliced cucumbers with squeeze of lemon juice and salt and pepper to taste (16 calories)

Dinner: one serving Stuffed Sweet Potato with Hummus Dressing (472 calories)

**WEEK 2**

DAY 8

Breakfast: one serving Muffin-Tin Quiches with Smoked Cheddar & Potato (238 calories)

A.M. Snack: one cup sliced cucumber with a squeeze of lemon juice and salt & pepper to taste (16 calories)

Lunch: one serving Stuffed Sweet Potato with Hummus Dressing (472 calories)

P.M. Snack: one plum (30 calories)

Dinner: one serving Roasted Root Veggies and Greens over Spiced Lentils (453 calories)

Meal-Prep Tip: Prepare one serving of Creamy Blueberry-Pecan Overnight Oatmeal to have for breakfast tomorrow

DAY 9

Breakfast: one serving Creamy Blueberry-Pecan Overnight Oatmeal (291 calories)

A.M. Snack: one cup red wine (85 calories)

Lunch: 1 serving Roasted Veggie and Quinoa Salad (351 calories)

P.M. Snack: one t two cup sliced cucumber with a pinch of salt and pepper (8 calories)

Dinner: one serving One-Skillet Salmon with Fennel and Sun-Dried Tomato Couscous (543 calories)

DAY 10

Breakfast: one serving Everything Bagel Avocado Toast with a side of one hard-boiled egg (250 calories)

A.M. Snack: one cup red wine (85 calories)

Lunch: one serving Roasted Veggie and Quinoa Salad (351 calories)

P.M. Snack: dark chocolate (230 calories)

Dinner: one serving Chickpea Quinoa Bowl (479 calories)

DAY 11

Breakfast: one serving Muesli with Raspberries (287 calories)

A.M. Snack: dark chocolate (230 calories)

Lunch: one serving Roasted Veggie and Quinoa Salad (351 calories)

P.M. Snack: red wine (85 calories)

Dinner: one serving Slow-Cooker Pasta e Fagioli Soup Freezer Pack (457 calories)

DAY 12

Breakfast: one serving Everything Bagel Avocado Toast with a side of 1 hard-boiled egg (250 calories)

A.M. Snack: one cup red wine (85 calories)

Lunch: one serving Roasted Veggie and Quinoa Salad (351 calories)

P.M. Snack: one cup nonfat plain Greek yogurt with one Tbsp. chopped walnuts (181 calories)

Dinner: one serving No-Noodle Eggplant Lasagna with two cups mixed greens topped with one Tbsp. Herb Vinaigrette (364 calories)

Meal-Prep Tip: Reserve one serving of the No-Noodle Eggplant Lasagna to have for lunch tomorrow.

DAY 13

Meal-Prep Tip: Start cooking the Slow-Cooker Chicken & Chickpea Soup in the morning so it's ready in time for dinner.

Breakfast: 1 serving Muesli with Redwine (287 calories)

A.M. Snack: dark chocolate (230 calories)

Lunch: one serving No-Noodle Eggplant Lasagna (301 calories)

P.M. Snack: one cup sliced red bell pepper with three Tbsp. hummus (106 calories)

Dinner: one serving Slow-Cooker Chicken & Chickpea Soup (446 calories)

Meal-Prep Tip: Reserve two servings of the Slow-Cooker Chicken & Chickpea Soup to have for lunch on Days 14 and 15.

DAY 14

Breakfast: one serving Everything Bagel Avocado Toast with a side of one hard-boiled egg (250 calories)

A.M. Snack: 1/2 cup red wine (85 calories)

Lunch: 1 serving Slow-Cooker Chicken and Chickpea Soup (446 calories)

P.M. Snack: one cup sliced cucumber with a pinch of salt and pepper (8 calories)

Dinner: one serving One-Pot Greek Pasta (487 calories)

**WEEK 3**

DAY 15

Breakfast: one serving Creamy Blueberry-Pecan Overnight Oatmeal (291 calories)

A.M. Snack: one cup red wine (85 calories)

Lunch: 1 serving Slow-Cooker Chicken & Chickpea Soup (446 calories)

P.M. Snack: dark chocolate (230 calories)

Dinner: one serving Summer Shrimp Salad with 2 cups mixed greens topped with one Tbsp. Parsley-Lemon Vinaigrette (394 calories)

DAY 16

Breakfast:one serving Muesli with Raspberries (287 calories)

A.M. Snack: one to two cup sliced cucumbers with a pinch of salt & pepper (8 calories)

Lunch: one serving Vegan Superfood Buddha Bowls (381 calories)

P.M. Snack: one to two cup sliced red bell pepper (14 calories)

Dinner: one serving Lemon Tahini Couscous with Chicken and Vegetables (528 calories)

DAY 17

Breakfast: one serving Muffin-Tin Quiches with Smoked Cheddar and Potato (238 calories)

A.M. Snack: one to two cup red wine (85 calories)

Lunch: one serving Vegan Superfood Buddha Bowl (381 calories)

P.M. Snack: one cup red wine (85 calories)

Dinner: one serving Walnut-Rosemary Crusted Salmon with one serving Easy Brown Rice Pilaf with Spring Vegetables (538 calories)

DAY 18

Breakfast: two servings Berry-Mint Kefir Smoothies (274 calories)

A.M. Snack: dark chocolate (230 calories)

Lunch: two serving Vegan Superfood Buddha Bowl (381 calories)

P.M. Snack: one to two cup nonfat plain Greek yogurt (66 calories)

Dinner: one serving Farfalle with Tuna, Lemon and Fennel with two cups mixed greens and one Tbsp. Parsley-Lemon Vinaigrette (460 calories)

DAY 19

Breakfast: one serving Muffin-Tin Quiches with Smoked Cheddarand Potato (238 calories)

A.M. Snack: one plum (30 calories)

Lunch: one serving Vegan Superfood Buddha Bowls (381 calories)

P.M. Snack: five oz. nonfat plain Greek yogurt with one cup blueberries (105 calories)

Dinner: one serving Cilantro Bean Burgers with Creamy Avocado-Lime Slaw with two cups mixed greens andone Tbsp. Parsley-Lemon Vinaigrette (472 calories)

DAY 20

Breakfast: two servings Berry-Mint Kefir Smoothies (274 calories)

A.M. Snack: two or three cup red wine (85 calories)

Lunch: one serving Mason Jar Power Salad with Chickpeas & Tuna (430 calories)

P.M. Snack: two to three cup red wine (85 calories)

Dinner: one serving Roasted Chicken and Winter Squash over Mixed Greens (415 calories)

DAY 21

Breakfast: two servings Berry-Mint Kefir Smoothies (274 calories)

A.M. Snack: one or two cup red wine (85 calories)

Lunch: one serving Mason Jar Power Salad with Chickpeas and Tuna (430 calories)

P.M. Snack: dark chocolate (230)

Dinner: one serving Sweet and Spicy Roasted Salmon with Wild Rice Pilaf with two cups mixed greens and one Tbsp. Parsley-Lemon Vinaigrette (443 calories)

Meal-Prep Tip: Reserve one serving of the Sweet and Spicy Roasted Salmon with Wild Rice Pilaf to have for lunch tomorrow.

## WEEK 4

DAY 22

Breakfast: one serving Pineapple Green Smoothie (297 calories)

A.M. Snack: dark chocolate (130 calories)

Lunch: one salmon fillet (left over from Sweet and Spicy Roasted Salmon with Wild Rice Pilaf) with one cup Roasted Butternut Squash and Root Vegetables and 1/3 cup Lemon-Roasted Mixed Vegetables (354 calories)

P.M. Snack: dark chocolate (230 calories)

Dinner: one serving Green Salad with Edamame and Beets topped with one of an avocado (405 calories)

DAY 23

Meal-Prep Tip: Start cooking the Slow-Cooker Pasta e Fagioli Soup Freezer Pack in the morning so it's ready in time for dinner.

Breakfast: 1 serving (287 calories)

A.M. Snack: dark chocolate (230 calories)

Lunch: one serving Piled-High Greek Vegetable Pitas (399 calories)

P.M. Snack: one cup sliced red bell pepper (29 calories)

Dinner: one serving Slow-Cooker Pasta e Fagioli Soup Freezer Pack (457 calories)


DAY 24

Breakfast: one serving Everything Bagel Avocado Toast with a side of 1 hard-boiled egg (250 calories)

A.M. Snack: two cup red wine (85 calories)

Lunch: one serving Piled-High Greek Vegetable Pitas (399 calories)

P.M. Snack: dark chocolate (230 calories)

Dinner: one serving Quinoa, Chicken and Broccoli Salad with Roasted Lemon Dressing (481 calories)

DAY 25

Breakfast: one serving Blueberry Almond Chia Pudding (229 calories)

A.M. Snack: five oz. nonfat plain Greek yogurt with 1/4 cup blueberries and one Tbsp. chopped walnuts (153 calories)

Lunch: one serving Piled-High Greek Vegetable Pitas (399 calories)

P.M. Snack: dark chocolate (230 calories)

Dinner: 1 serving  Cod with Roasted Tomatoes and 3/4 cup Quinoa Avocado Salad (364 calories)

DAY 26

Breakfast: one serving Everything Bagel Avocado Toast with a side of 1 hard-boiled egg (250 calories)

A.M. Snack: one cup red wine (85 calories)

Lunch: 1 serving Piled-High Greek Vegetable Pitas (399 calories)

P.M. Snack: five oz. nonfat plain Greek yogurt with 1/3 cup blackberries (104 calories)

Dinner: serving Caprese Stuffed Portobello Mushrooms with three cup Quinoa Avocado Salad (393 calories)

DAY 27

Breakfast: one serving Muesli with Raspberries (287 calories)

A.M. Snack: dark chocolate (230 calories)

Lunch: one serving Instant Pot White Chicken Chili Freezer Pack with one cup blueberries (298 calories)

P.M. Snack: three cup sliced red bell pepper with one Tbsp. hummus (47 calories)

Dinner: one serving Stuffed Eggplant with one serving Traditional Greek Salad (513 calories)


DAY 28

Breakfast: two servings Berry-Mint Kefir Smoothies (274 calories)

A.M. Snack: one cup sliced red bell pepper (14 calories)

Lunch: one serving Instant Pot White Chicken Chili Freezer Pack with one cup blueberries (298 calories)

P.M. Snack: one cup sliced cucumbers with a pinch of salt and pepper (8 calories)

Dinner: one serving Chickpea Pasta with Lemony-Parsley Pesto (630 calories)


**WEEK 5**

DAY 29

Breakfast: one serving Everything Bagel Avocado Toast with a side of one hard-boiled egg (250 calories)

A.M. Snack: two cup fresh raspberries with five walnut halves (108 calories)

Lunch: one serving Instant Pot White Chicken Chili Freezer Pack with one cup blueberries (298 calories)

P.M. Snack: two cup red wine with seven walnut halves (132 calories)

Dinner: one serving Greek Roasted Fish with Vegetables (422 calories)

DAY 30

Meal-Prep Tip: Start cooking the Slow-Cooker Mediterranean Chicken and Orzo in the morning so it's ready in time for dinner.

Breakfast: one serving Blueberry Almond Chia Pudding (229 calories)

A.M. Snack: dark chocolate (230 calories)

Lunch: one serving Instant Pot White Chicken Chili Freezer Pack with one cup red wine (298 calories)

P.M. Snack: twelve walnut halves (157 calories)

Dinner: one serving Slow-Cooker Chicken & Orzo with 1 serving Cucumber, Tomato & Avocado Salad (450 calories)

# Chapter 9: SIRTFOOD RECIPES

*1.Heated Potatoes with Spicy Chickpea Stew*

Nutrition: Calories: 322 kcal Protein: 8.08 g Fat: 5.97 g Sugars: 61.85 g

Ingredients

• 4-6 heating potatoes, pricked all more than 2 tablespoons olive oil

• 2 red onions, finely cut

• 4 cloves garlic, ground or squashed 2cm ginger, ground

• 2 tablespoons unsweetened cocoa powder (or cacao)

• 2 x 400g tins chickpeas (or kidney beans if you like) including the chickpea water DON'T DRAIN!!

• 2 yellow peppers (or whatever color you like!), cut into reduced down pieces 2 tablespoons parsley in addition to extra for decorating

• Salt and pepper to taste (discretionary)

• Side salad

• ½ - 2 teaspoons chili pieces (contingent upon how hot you like things) 2 tablespoons cumin seeds

• 2 tablespoons turmeric

• Sprinkle of water

• 2 x 400g tins cleaved tomatoes

Directions

a. Preheat the oven to 200C.

b. Then set up the various ingredients.

c. At the point when the oven is sufficiently hot, at that point put your preparing potatoes in the oven. Cook for 60 minutes.

d. When the potatoes are in the oven, at that point place the olive oil and sliced red onion in an enormous wide pot. Cook it tenderly, with the cover on for 5 minutes. Keep cooking until the onions are delicate yet not earthy colored.

e. Remove the top. Include the garlic, ginger, cumin, and chili. Presently cook for a moment on low warmth. At that point include the turmeric and a minuscule sprinkle of water and cook for one moment. Take care that the dish gets excessively dry.

f. Presently include the tomatoes, cocoa powder (or cacao), chickpeas (additionally incorporate the chickpea water). Likewise, add yellow pepper and bring to boil. Stew on a low warmth for around 45 minutes. Thus the sauce is thick (however don't allow it to consume!).

g. The stew ought to be cooked generally simultaneously as the potatoes.

h. At long last, mix in the two tablespoons of parsley, and some salt and pepper if you wish. At last, serve the stew on the prepared potatoes.

## 2.Greek Salad Skewers

Nourishment:  Calories: 287 kcal  Protein: 19.5 g  Fat: 17.45 g
Starches: 14.84 g

Ingredients
• 2 wooden sticks, absorbed water for 30 minutes before utilize
8 huge dark olives
• 1 yellow pepper, cut into eight squares
• ½ red onion, sliced down the middle and isolated into eight
pieces 100g (about 10cm) cucumber, cut into four cuts and
split 100g feta, cut into 8 cubes
• 8 cherry tomatoes

For the dressing
• 1 tbsp additional virgin olive oil Juice of ½ lemon
•1 tsp balsamic vinegar
• Hardly any leaves oregano (finely cut)
• liberal flavoring of salt and ground dark pepper
• ½ clove garlic, stripped and squashed
• Barely any leaves of basil, finely sliced (or ½ tsp dried
blended herbs to supplant basil and oregano)

Directions
As a matter of first importance string each stick with the salad
ingredients in the accompanying request: - Olive, Tomato,

Yellow pepper, Red onion, Cucumber, Feta, Tomato, Olive, Yellow pepper, Red onion, Cucumber, and Feta.

Presently place all the dressing ingredients in a little bowl. Combine and pour over the sticks.

### 3.Kale, Edamame and Tofu Curry

Nourishment:  Calories: 407 kcal  Protein: 27.67 g  Fat: 9.98 g
Starches: 57.95 g

Ingredients
- 1 tbsp rapeseed oil
- 1 huge onion, cleaved
- 4 cloves garlic, stripped and ground
- 4 .1 huge thumb (7cm) new ginger, stripped and ground 1 red chili, deseeded and meagerly cut
- 50g solidified soya beans
- 200g firm tofu, sliced into solid shapes 2 tomatoes, generally cut
- Juice of 1 lime
- 200g kale leaves, stalks removed and torn
- 1/2 tsp ground turmeric
- 1/4 tsp cayenne pepper 1 tsp paprika
- 1/2 tsp ground cumin 1 tsp salt
- 250g dried red lentils 1 liter boiling water

Directions
a. Put the oil in a substantial bottomed pan. Cook over low to medium warmth. Include the onion in it and cook for 5 minutes.
b. At that point include the garlic, ginger, and chili. After including them and cook for two minutes.

c. Include turmeric, cayenne, paprika, cumin, and salt. Mix through before you include the red lentils. Mix once more.

d. Pour in the boiling water. Boil for 10 minutes. Presently lessen the warmth and cook for a further 20-30 minutes until the curry has a thick '•porridge' consistency.

Include the soya beans, tofu, and tomatoes, cook for 5 minutes more. Include the lime juice and kale leaves. Cook until the Kale is simply delicate.

## 4.Sirt Food Miso-Marinated Cod with Stir-Fried Greens and Sesame

Nutrition: Calories: 355 kcal  Protein: 40.31 g  Fat: 10.87 g Sugars: 25.94 g

Ingredients
- 20g miso
- 1 tbsp mirin
- 1 tbsp additional virgin olive oil 200g skinless cod filet 20g red onion, cut
- 1 tsp sesame seeds
- 5g parsley, generally cleaved 1 tbsp tamari
- 30g buckwheat
- 1 tsp ground turmeric
- 40g celery, cut
- one garlic clove, finely cleaved one superior stew, finely sliced 1 tsp cut new ginger 60g green beans
- 50g Kale, generally cleaved

Directions
Here you write about how to do the recipe like:
a.  insert 1 kg of flou and 2 eggs in a container;
b.  cook about 50 minutes
c.  enjoy your dish!

## 5.Chocolate Bark

Nutrition: Protein: 20.7 g  Calories: 523 kcal  Fat: 40.76 g Sugars: 26.65 g

Ingredients
- 1 slight strip orange
- ¾ cup pistachio nuts, cooked, chilled and sliced into huge pieces
- 1 cardamom unit, finely squashed and sieved
- 12 ounces (340 g) tempered, without dairy dark chocolate (65% cocoa content) 2 teaspoons flaky ocean salt
- Candy or candy thermometer
- ¼ cup hazelnuts, toasted, chilled, stripped and cleaved into huge pieces
- ¼ cup pumpkin seeds, toasted and chilled 1 tablespoon chia seeds
- 1 tablespoon sesame seeds, toasted and cooled 1 teaspoon ground orange strip

Directions
a. Preheat the oven to 100-150 ° F (66 ° C). Line a preparing sheet with material paper.
b. Finely cut the orange across and place it on the readied preparing sheet. Prepare for 2 to 3 hours until dry yet marginally sticky. Remove it from the oven and let it cool.

c.  At the point when they sufficiently cool to deal with them, cut the orange cuts into parts; put them in a safe place.

d.  In an enormous bowl, blend the nuts, seeds, and ground orange strip until joined. Place the blend in a single layer on a preparing sheet fixed with kitchen material. Put it in a safe place.

e.  Melt the chocolate in a water shower until it arrives at 88 to 90 ° F (32 to 33 ° C) and pours it over the nut blend to cover it.

f.  At the point when the chocolate is semi-cold yet at the same time sticky, sprinkle the surface with ocean salt and bits of orange.

Place the blend in a chilly zone of your kitchen or refrigerate until the outside layer cools totally, and cut it into reduced down pieces.

## 6. Salmon and Spinach Quiche

Nourishment: Calories: 903 kcal  Protein: 65.28 g  Fat: 59.79 g  Starches: 30.79 g

Ingredients
- 600 g solidified leaf spinach 1 clove of garlic
- 1 onion
- 50 g spread
- 200 g sharp cream 3 eggs
- Salt, pepper, nutmeg 1 pack of puff cake
- 150 g solidified salmon filets 200 g smoked salmon
- 1 little Bunch of dill 1 untreated lemon

Directions
a.  Allow the spinach to defrost and crush well.
b.  Strip the garlic and onion and cut into fine 3D squares. Cut the salmon filet into solid shapes 1-1.5 cm thick. Cut the smoked salmon into strips.
c.  Wash the dill, pat dry, and cut.
d.  Wash the lemon with boiling water, dry, rub the get-up-and-go finely with a kitchen grater, and crush the lemon.
e.  Warmth the margarine in a dish. Sweat the garlic and onion solid shapes in it for approx. 2-3 minutes.
f.  Include spinach and sweat quickly.
g.  Include sharp cream, lemon juice and pizzazz, eggs and dill and blend well. Season with salt, pepper, and nutmeg.

h. Preheat the oven to 200 degrees top/base warmth (180 degrees convection).

i. Oil a springform container and reveal the puff baked good in it and pull up anxious. Prick the dough with a fork (so it doesn't rise excessively).

j. Pour in the spinach and egg blend and smooth out. Spread salmon 3D shapes and smoked salmon strips on top.

The quiche in the oven (network, center inset) around 30-40 min. Yellow gold prepare.

## 7.Turmeric Chicken and Kale Salad with Honey Lime Dressing

Nutrition: Calories: 1290 kcal Protein: 131.39 g Fat: 66.95 g Sugars: 40.87 g

Ingredients

For chicken

• 1 teaspoon ghee or 1 tablespoon of coconut oil

• ½ medium brown onion, diced

• 250-300 g/9 oz. Ground chicken or cubed chicken thighs 1 huge clove of garlic, finely diced

• 1 teaspoon turmeric powder 1 teaspoon lime pizzazz

• ½ lime juice

• ½ tsp salt + pepper For salad

• 6 stems of broccoli or 2 cups of broccoli florets 2 tablespoons of pumpkin seeds

• 3 tbsp lime juice

• 1 diced or ground a little bit of garlic 3 tablespoons additional virgin olive oil

• 1 tsp crude nectar

• 1/2 teaspoon entire grain 1/2 teaspoon ocean salt Pepper

• 3 enormous kale leaves, stems evacuated and cut

• ½Avocado, cut

• A bunch of new coriander leaves, cleaved A bunch of new parsley leaves cut dressing

Directions

a. In a little pan, heat the ghee or coconut oil over medium to high warmth. Include the onion and sauté for 4-5 minutes on medium warmth, until brilliant. Connect the vile chicken and garlic and twirl over medium-high warmth for 2-3 minutes, breaking it separated.

b. Connect the turmeric, lime get-up-and-go, lime juice, salt, and pepper and cook for a further 3-4 minutes, mixing as often as possible. Put aside the cooked slush.

c. Carry a little pan of water to boil while the chicken cooks. Mix in the broccolini and cook 2 minutes. Wash under virus water, and slice into three to four pieces each.

d. Toss the pumpkin seeds from the chicken into the pan and toast for 2 minutes over medium warmth, blending now and again to forestall consuming. Season to a touch of salt. Store aside. Crude pumpkin seeds ought to likewise be utilized well.

e. In a salad bowl, place the cut kale, and pour over the dressing. Hurl the kale with the sauce, and rub it with your palms. This will mollify the kale, sort of like what citrus juice never really fish or meat it' cooks' it a tad.

The cooked rice, broccolini, new herbs, pumpkin seeds, and cuts of avocado are in the long run hurled.

## 8.Buckwheat Noodles with Chicken Kale and Miso Dressing

Nutrition: Calories: 256 kcal Protein: 10.82 g Fat: 8.95 g Sugars: 37.03 g

Ingredients

For Noodles

• 2-3 bunches of kale leaves (removed from the stem and generally cut) Buckwheat noodles 150 g/5 oz (100% buckwheat, no wheat)

• 1 medium unfenced chicken bosom, cut or cubed 1 long red chili, meagerly cut

• 2 large garlic cloves, finely diced

• 2-3 tablespoons of Tamari sauce (sans gluten soy sauce)

• 3-4 shiitake mushrooms, cut into cuts 1 teaspoon of coconut oil or ghee

• 1 brown onion, finely diced

For miso dressing

• 1½ tbsp new natural miso 1 tbsp Tamari sauce

• 1 tablespoon of additional virgin olive oil 1 tablespoon lemon or lime juice

• 1 teaspoon sesame oil

Directions

a. Bring a medium pot of boiling water. Connect the kale and cook until marginally shriveled, for 1 moment. Remove and put in a safe place, at that point take the water back to the boil. Include the soba noodles and cook (normally around 5 minutes) as indicated by bundling directions. Put in a safe place and flush under virus water.

b. In the interim, in a little ghee or coconut oil (about a teaspoon), sauté the shiitake mushrooms for 2-3 minutes, until gently seared on either side. Sprinkle with salt from the ocean, and put in a safe place.

c. Warmth more coconut oil or ghee in a similar pan over medium to high warmth. Mix in onion and chili for 2-3 minutes, at that point include bits of chicken. Cook over medium warmth for 5 minutes, blending a couple of times, at that point include the garlic, tamari sauce, and some sprinkle of water. Cook for another 2-3 minutes, continually mixing until chicken is cooked through.

d. In the end, include the kale and soba noodles and warm up by blending through the food.

e. Directly toward the finish of the cooking, blend the miso dressing and shower over the noodles, so you'll keep each one of those helpful probiotics alive and dynamic.

## 9.Asian King Prawn Stir-Fry with Buckwheat Noodles

Nutrition:  Calories: 251 kcal  Protein: 22.97 g  Fat: 3.71 g
Sugars: 34.14 g

Ingredients
• 150g crude illustrious shrimps in shelled skins
• 2 teaspoons of tamari (you can utilize soy sauce if you don't evade gluten) 2 teaspoons additional virgin olive oil
• 1 teaspoon of finely sliced new ginger 20g red onion, cut into cuts
• 40g celery, cut and cut into cuts
• 75g cut green beans 50g kale, coarsely sliced 100 ml of chicken stock
• 5g lovage or celery leaves
• 75g soba (buckwheat noodles)
• 1 clove of garlic, finely sliced
• 1 flying perspective on finely sliced stew

Directions
a. Warmth a griddle over high warmth, at that point cook the prawns for 2–3 minutes in 1 teaspoon tamari and 1 teaspoon oil. Put the prawns on a plate. Wipe the work out with paper from the oven, as you will utilize it once more.
b. Cook the noodles 5–8 minutes in boiling water, or as demonstrated on the parcel. Channel and set aside.

c.  In the meantime, over medium-high warmth, fry the garlic, stew, and ginger, red onion, celery, beans, and kale in the rest of the oil for 2–3 minutes. Remove the stock and bring to the boil, at that point cook for a couple of minutes until the vegetables are cooked yet crunchy.

d.  Include the prawns, noodles, and leaves of lovage/celery to the pan, take back to the boil, at that point evacuate the warmth and serve.

## 10.Choc Chip Granola

Nutrition: Calories: 914 kcal  Protein: 40.19 g  Fat: 63.05 g
Starches: 88.74 g

Ingredients
- 200g enormous oat pieces Roughly 50 g walnut nuts cut
- 2 tbsp rice syrup
- 60 g of good quality (70%) dark chocolate shavings
- 3 tablespoons of light olive oil 20g margarine
- 1 tablespoon of dark brown sugar

Directions
a. Oven preheats to 160 ° C (140 ° C fan/Gas 3). Line an enormous heating plate with a sheet of silicone or material for preparing.
b. In an enormous bowl, join the oats and walnuts. Warmth the olive oil, margarine, brown sugar, and rice malt syrup tenderly in a little non-stick pan until the spread has melted, and the sugar and syrup break up. Try not to let boil. Pour the syrup over the oats and mix completely until completely secured with the oats.
c. Spread the granola over the heating plate and spread directly into the corners. Leave the blend bunches with separating, rather than spreading. Heat for 20 minutes in the oven until brilliant brown is simply tinged at the edges.

Remove from the oven, and leave totally to cool on the plate.

d. At the point when chilly, split with your fingers any bigger bumps on the plate and afterward blend them in the chocolate chips. Put the granola in a hermetically sealed tube or container, or pour it. The granola is to keep going for in any event fourteen days.

*11.Sweet-smelling Chicken Breast, Kale, Red Onion, and Salsa*

Nutrition: Calories: 149 kcal, Protein: 15.85 g, Fat: 5.09 g, Sugars: 10.53 g

Ingredients
- 120g skinless, boneless chicken bosom 2 teaspoons ground turmeric
- 20g red onion, cut
- 1 teaspoon new ginger, sliced 50g buckwheat
- ¼ lemon
- 1 tablespoon extra-virgin olive oil 50g kale, cleaved

Directions
a. To set up the salsa, remove the tomato eye and finely cut. Include the chili, parsley, capers, lemon juice, and blend.
b. Preheat the oven to 220°C. Pour 1 teaspoon of the turmeric, the lemon juice and a little oil on the chicken bosom and marinate. Permit to remain for 5–10 minutes.
c. Place an ovenproof griddle on the warmth and cook the marinated chicken for a moment on each side to accomplish a pale brilliant color. At that point move the container containing the chicken to the oven and permit to remain for 8–10 minutes or until it is finished. Remove from the oven and spread with foil, put in a safe place for 5 minutes before serving.

d. Put the kale in a liner and cook for 5 minutes. Pour a little oil in a pan and fry the red onions and the ginger to turn out to be delicate yet not shaded. Include the cooked kale and keep on frying for another minute.

Cook the buckwheat adhering to the bundle's guidelines utilizing the rest of the turmeric. Serve close by the chicken, salsa, and vegetables.

*12.Kale and Red Onion Dhal with Buckwheat*

Nutrition:

Calories: 355 kcal, Protein: 14.39 g, Fat: 5.7 g, Sugars: 63.41 g

Ingredients

- *½ tablespoon olive oil*
- *½ little red onion, cut 1 ½ garlic cloves, squashed 1cm ginger, ground*
- *100ml water*
- *50g kale or spinach*
- *80g buckwheat or brown rice*
- *½ flying creatures eye chili, deseeded and finely cleaved 1 teaspoon turmeric*
- *1 teaspoon garam masala 80g red lentils*
- *200ml coconut milk ....*

Directions

a. Warmth up the olive oil, include the cut onion, and cook on a low warmth for 5 minutes until relaxed with the top on. At that point, include the ginger, garlic, and chili and keep cooking for an additional 1 moment.

b. Add to it, the garam masala, turmeric, and a sprinkle of water. Cook for 1 increasingly minute before including the coconut milk, red lentils, and 200ml water.

c. Altogether combine all and cook over a delicate warmth for 20 minutes with the top shut. At the point when the dhal begins staying, include somewhat more water and mix once in a while.

d. Include the kale, following 20 minutes and completely mix and still spread the cover to cook for an extra 5 minutes or 1-2 minutes when you substitute with spinach.

e. Put the buckwheat in a pan and pour boiling water like 15 minutes before the curry prepares. Permit the water to boil and cook for 10-12 minutes. Channel the buckwheat and present with the dhal.

*13.Chargrilled Beef, A Red Wine Jus, Onion Rings, Garlic Kale, And Herb Roasted Potatoes*

Nutrition: Calories: 244 kcal   Protein: 14.26 g   Fat: 14.46 g Sugars: 14.69 g

Ingredients

- *100g potatoes, stripped and dice*
- *1 tablespoon extra-virgin olive oil*
- *120–150g x 3.5cm-thick hamburger filet steak 40ml red wine 150ml meat stock*
- *1 teaspoon tomato purée 1 teaspoon cornflour*
- *1 tablespoon water*
- *5g parsley, finely cleaved*
- *50g red onion, cut into rings 50g kale, cut*
- *1 garlic clove, finely cleaved ....*

Directions

a. Preheat the oven to 220°C and place the potatoes in boiling water and cook for 4–5 minutes, channel. Pour 1 teaspoon oil in a simmering tin and meal the potatoes for 35–45 minutes turning the potatoes on each side like clockwork to guarantee they cook equitably.

b. Remove from the oven when completely cooked, sprinkle with cut parsley, and blend all together.

c.  Pour 1 teaspoon of the oil on a pan and fry the onion for 5-7 minutes to turn out to be delicate and conveniently caramelized. Keep it warm.

d.  Place the kale in a pan, steam for 2–3 minutes, and channel. In ½ teaspoon of oil, fry the garlic for 1 moment to turn out to be delicate however not hued. Add the kale and keep on singing for an additional 1–2 minutes to get delicate. Keep up the glow.

e.  Over high warmth, place an ovenproof pan until it gets smoking. At that point utilize the ½ a teaspoon of the oil to cover the meat and fry over a medium-high warmth. Remove the meat and put aside to rest.

f.  Pour the wine to the hot pan and air pocket to reduce the wine amount significantly to shape sweet and to have a concentrated flavor. Include the tomato purée and stock to the steak container and boil. Include the cornflour paste little at once to go about as a thickener to until the ideal consistency is accomplished. Include any juices from the refreshed steak and present with the kale, onion rings, cooked potatoes, and red wine sauce.

*14.Braised Leek With Pine Nuts*

Nutrition: Calories: 95 kcal Protein: 1.35 g Fat: 4.84 g Sugars: 12.61 g

Ingredients

- *20 g Ghee*
- *1 tablespoon new oregano*
- *tablespoon Pine nuts (simmered)*
- *2 teaspoon Olive oil 2 pieces Leek*
- *150 ml Vegetable stock new parsley ....*

Directions

a. Cut the leek into thin rings and finely slice the herbs. Cook the pine nuts in a dry pan over medium warmth.
b. Melt the ghee along with the olive oil in a huge pan.
c. Cook the leek until brilliant brown for 5 minutes, blending continually.
d. Include the vegetable stock and cook for an additional 10 minutes until the leek is delicate. Mix in the herbs and sprinkle the pine nuts on the dish not long before serving.

## 15.Prepared Pan With Cashew Nuts

Nourishment:  Calories: 573 kcal  Protein: 15.25 g Fat: 27.81 g Starches: 77.91 g

Ingredients

- 150 g Pak choi
- 2 tablespoon Coconut oil 2 pieces Red onion
- 2 pieces yellow chime pepper 250 g White cabbage
- 50 g Mung bean grows 4 pieces Pineapple cuts 50 g Cashew nuts

For the prepared sauce:

- 60 ml Apple juice vinegar
- 1 teaspoon Coconut-Aminos 2 teaspoon Arrowroot powder 75 ml Water
- 4 tablespoon Coconut bloom sugar 1½ tablespoon Tomato paste ....

Directions

a. Generally cut the vegetables.
b. Blend the bolt root with five tablespoons of cold water into a paste.
c. At that point put the various elements for the sauce in a pan and include the arrowroot paste for official.
d. Melt the coconut oil in a container and fry the onion.

e. Include the ringer pepper, cabbage, pak choi and bean sprouts and sautéed food until the vegetables become somewhat milder.

f. Include the pineapple and cashew nuts and mix a couple of more occasions.

g. Pour a little sauce over the wok dish and serve.

## 16. Dish With Spinach And Eggplant

Nutrition: Calories: 446 kcal  Protein: 13.95 g  Fat: 31.82 g
Sugars: 30.5 g

Ingredients

- *Olive oil 3 tablespoon*
  *Spinach (new) 450 g*
  *Tomatoes 4 pieces*
- *Egg 2 pieces*
- *1 piece Eggplant*
- *2 teaspoons Lemon juice*
- *4 tablespoon Almond flour*
- *2 pieces Onion*
- *60 ml Almond milk*

Directions

a. Preheat the oven to 200 ° C.

b. Cut the eggplants, onions, and tomatoes into cuts and sprinkle salt on the eggplant cuts.

c. Brush the eggplants and onions with olive oil and fry them in a barbecue pan. Shrink the spinach in an enormous pan over moderate warmth and channel in a sifter.

d. Put the vegetables in layers in a lubed heating dish: first the eggplants, at that point the spinach and afterward the onion and the tomato. Repeat this.

e. Whisk eggs with almond milk, lemon juice, salt, and pepper and pour over the vegetables.

f. Sprinkle almond flour over the dish and heat in the oven for around 30 to 40 minute

## 17. Veggie Lover Paleo Ratatouille

Nourishment:  Calories: 273 kcal  Protein: 5.66 g  Fat: 14.49 g Starches: 35.81 g

Ingredients

- 200 g Tomato solid shapes (can) 1/2 pieces Onion
- 2 cloves Garlic
- 1 piece hot peppers
- 1 teaspoon dried thyme
- 1/4 teaspoon dried oregano
- 1/4 TL Chili drops 2 tablespoon Olive oil 1 piece Eggplant
- 1 piece Zucchini

Directions

a. Preheat the oven to 180 ° C and gently oil a round or oval shape. Finely slice the onion and garlic.

b. Blend the tomato shapes with garlic, onion, oregano and stew chips, season with salt and pepper, and put on the base of the preparing dish.

c. Utilize a mandolin, a cheese slicer or a sharp blade to cut the eggplant, zucchini and hot pepper into dainty cuts.

d. Put the vegetables in a bowl (make hovers, start at the edge and work inside).

e. Shower the staying olive oil on the vegetables and sprinkle with thyme, salt, and pepper.

f. Spread the preparing dish with a bit of material paper and heat in the oven for 45 to 55 minutes.

## 18.Courgette And Broccoli Soup

Nutrition:   Calories: 178 kcal   Protein: 5.7 g   Fat: 14.43 g
Sugars: 10.57 g

Ingredients

- 2 tablespoon Coconut oil 1 piece Red onion
- 1 piece Zucchini
- •750 ml Vegetable stock
- 2 cloves Garlic
- 300 g Broccoli

Directions

a. Finely slice the onion and garlic, cut the broccoli into florets, and the zucchini into cuts.
b. Melt the coconut oil in a soup pot and fry the onion with the garlic. Cook the zucchini for a couple of moments.
c. Include broccoli and vegetable stock and stew for around 5 minutes. Puree the soup with a hand blender and season with salt and pepper.

## 19. Frittata With Spring Onions And Asparagus

Nourishment: Calories: 464 kcal  Protein: 24.23 g  Fat: 37.84 g  Starches: 7.33 g

Ingredients

- 5 pieces Egg
- 100 g Asparagus tips 4 pieces Spring onions 1 teaspoon Tarragon
- 1 juice Chili drops
- 80 ml Almond milk
- 2 tablespoon Coconut oil 1 clove Garlic

Directions

a. Preheat the oven to 220 ° C.
b. Crush the garlic and finely slice the spring onions.
c. Whisk the eggs with the almond milk and season with salt and pepper.
d. Melt 1 tablespoon of coconut oil in a medium-sized cast iron dish and quickly fry the onion and garlic with the asparagus.
e. Remove the vegetables from the container and liquefy the rest of the coconut oil in the dish.
f. Pour in the egg blend and half of the whole vegetable.
g. Place the pan in the oven for 15 minutes until the egg has cemented.

h. At that point remove the pan from the oven and pour the remainder of the egg with the vegetables into the container.

i. Place the pan in the oven again for 15 minutes until the egg is overall quite free. Sprinkle the tarragon and chili drops on the dish before serving.

## 20.Cucumber Salad with Lime and Coriander

Nourishment: Calories: 57 kcal   Protein: 2 g   Fat: 0.41 g
Starches: 13.22 g

Ingredients

- *1 piece Red onion 2 pieces Cucumber*
- *2 tablespoon new coriander*
- *2 pieces Lime (juice)*

Directions

a. Cut the onion into rings and daintily cut the cucumber. Slice the coriander finely.
b. Place the onion rings in a bowl and season with about a large portion of a tablespoon of salt. Focus on it well and afterward fill the bowl with water.
c. Pour off the water and afterward flush the onion rings completely (in a strainer).
d. Set up the cucumber cuts with onion, lime juice, coriander, and olive oil in a salad bowl and mix everything great.
e. Season with somewhat salt.
f. You can keep this dish in the cooler in a secured bowl for a couple of days.

## 21.Kale and Feta Salad with Cranberry Dressing

Nourishment: Calories: 706 kcal  Protein: 15.62 g  Fat: 45.92 g Starches: 70.28 g

Ingredients

- 9oz kale, finely sliced 2oz walnuts, cleaved 3oz feta cheese, disintegrated
- 1 apple, stripped, cored and cut
- 4 Medjool dates, sliced
- For the Dressing 3oz cranberries
- ½ red onion, sliced 3 tablespoons olive oil 3 tablespoons water
- 2 teaspoons nectar
- 1 tablespoon red wine vinegar Sea salt

Direction

- Place the elements for the dressing into a food processor and procedure until smooth. If it appears to be too thick you can include some additional water if important. Place all the elements for the salad into a bowl. Pour on the dressing and hurl the salad until it is all around covered in the blend.

## 22.Fish, Egg and Caper Salad

Nutrition:  Calories: 309 kcal  Protein: 26.72 g  Fat: 12.23 g
Sugars: 25.76 g

Ingredients

- 1 tablespoon escapades
- 2 tablespoons garlic vinaigrette
- 2 hard-boiled eggs, stripped and quartered
- 3½ozred chicory or yellow if not accessible 5oz tinned fish drops in saline solution, depleted
- 3 ½ oz cucumber 1oz rocket arugula 6 pitted dark olives
- 2 tomatoes, cut
- 2 tablespoons new parsley, cut 1 red onion, sliced
- 1 stem of celery

Directions

- Place the fish, cucumber, olives, tomatoes, onion, chicory, celery, parsley and rocket arugula into a bowl. Pour in the vinaigrette and prepare the salad in the dressing. Serve onto plates and disperse the eggs and escapades on top.

### 23.Strawberry Buckwheat Pancakes

Nourishment:  Calories: 180 kcal  Protein: 7.46 g  Fat: 7.5 g
Starches: 22.58 g

Ingredients
- *3½oz strawberries, cleaved 3½ oz buckwheat flour*
- *1 teaspoon olive oil*
- *1 teaspoon olive oil for fricasseeing Freshly crushed juice of 1 orange*
- *1 egg*
- *8fl oz milk*

Directions
  a. Empty the milk into a bowl and blend in the egg and a teaspoon of olive oil. Filter in the flour to the fluid blend until smooth and velvety. Permit it to rest for 15 minutes. Warmth a little oil in a dish and pour in a fourth of the blend or to the size you like.
  b. Sprinkle in a fourth of the strawberries into the hitter. Cook for around 2 minutes on each side. Serve hot with a sprinkle of juice orange. You could have a go at exploring different avenues regarding different berries, for example, blueberries and blackberries.

## 24. Flapjacks with Apples and Blackcurrants

Nutrition: Calories: 470 kcal Protein: 11.71 g Fat: 16.83 g Sugars: 79 g

Ingredients

- 2 apples, cut into little pieces 2 cups of fast cooking oats
- 1 cup flour of your decision 1 tsp preparing powder
- 2 egg whites
- 1 ¼ cups of milk or soy/rice/coconut 2 tsp additional virgin olive oil
- A scramble of salt
- 2 tbsp. crude sugar, coconut sugar, or 2 tbsp. nectar that is warm and simple to appropriate

*For the berry beating:*

- *1 cup blackcurrants, washed and follows evacuated 3 tbsp. water may utilize less*
- *2 tbsp. sugar see above for types*

Directions

a. Place the elements for the garnish in a little pot stew, mixing now and again for around 10 minutes until it cooks down and the juices are discharged.
b. Take the dry ingredients and blend in a bowl. After, include the apples and the milk a piece at a time you may not utilize everything), until it is a hitter. Firmly whisk the egg

whites and afterward tenderly blend them into the hotcake player. Put aside in the cooler.

c. Pour a one-fourth of the oil onto a level dish or level frying pan, and when hot, empty a portion of the player into it in a flapjack shape. At the point when the flapjacks begin to have brilliant brown edges and structure air boils, they might be prepared to be tenderly flipped.

d. Test to be certain the base can live away from the dish before really flipping. Repeat for the following three hotcakes. Top every flapjack with the berries.

*25.Miso Caramelized Tofu*

Nutrition: Calories: 101 kcal  Protein: 4.22 g  Fat: 4.7 g Sugars: 12.38 g

Ingredients
- *35g buckwheat*
- *1 tsp ground turmeric*
- *2 tsp additional virgin olive oil 1 tsp tamari (or soy sauce)*
- *1 superior stew*
- *1 tbsp mirin 20g miso paste*
- *1 \* 150g firm tofu 40g celery, cut 35g red onion*
- *120g courgette*
- *1 garlic clove, finely cut*
- *1 tsp finely cut new ginger 50g kale, sliced*
- *2 tsp sesame seeds*

Directions
a. Pre-heat your over to 200C or gas mark 6. Spread a plate with heating material.
b. Join the mirin and miso together. Shakers the tofu and coat it in the mirin-miso blend in a resealable plastic sack. Put aside to marinate.
c. Slice the vegetables (aside from the kale) at a slanting point to create long cuts. Utilizing a liner, cook for the kale for 5 minutes and put in a safe place.

d. Scatter the tofu over the fixed plate and trimming with sesame seeds. Cook for 20 minutes, or until caramelized.

e. Wash the buckwheat utilizing running water and a sifter. Add to a container of boiling water close by turmeric and cook the buckwheat as per the bundle directions.

f. Warmth the oil in a pan over high warmth. Hurl in the vegetables, herbs, and flavors at that point fry for 2-3 minutes. Reduce to a medium warmth and fry for a further 5 minutes or until cooked yet at the same time crunchy.

## 26. Sirtfood Cauliflower Couscous and Turkey Steak

Nourishment: Calories: 462 kcal  Protein: 16.81 g  Fat: 39.86 g  Starches: 9.94 g

Ingredients

- 150g cauliflower, generally cut 1 garlic clove, finely sliced
- 2 tsp ground turmeric
- 30g sun-dried tomatoes, finely sliced 10g parsley
- 150g turkey steak 1 tsp dried sage Juice of ½ lemon 1 tbsp tricks
- 40g red onion, finely cut
- 1 bird's eye chili, finely sliced 1 tsp cleaved new ginger 2 tbsp additional virgin olive oil

Directions

a. Deteriorate the cauliflower utilizing a food processor. Mix in 1-2 heartbeats until the cauliflower has a breadcrumb-like consistency.

b. In a pan, fry garlic, stew, ginger, and red onion in 1 tsp olive oil for 2-3 minutes. Toss in the turmeric and cauliflower at that point cook for another 1-2 minutes. Remove from warmth and include the tomatoes and generally a large portion of the parsley.

c. Embellishment the turkey steak with wise and dress with oil. In a pan, over medium warmth, fry the turkey steak for

5 minutes, turning incidentally. When the steak is cooked include lemon juice, tricks, and a scramble of water. Mix and present with the couscous.

*27.Fish Salad*

Nourishment: Calories: 308 kcal  Protein: 27.13 g  Fat: 12.2 g
Starches: 24.6 g

Ingredients

- *100g red chicory*
- *2 hard-boiled eggs, stripped and quartered 2 tomatoes, cleaved*
- *2 tbsp new parsley, cleaved 1 red onion, cut*
- *150g fish pieces in brackish water, depleted 100g cucumber*
- *1 celery stem*
- *1 tbsp tricks*
- *2tbsp garlic vinaigrette*
- *25g rocket*
- *6 kalamata olives, pitted*

Directions

- Consolidate all ingredients in a bowl and serve.

## 28. Tofu and Shiitake Mushroom Soup

Nourishment:  Calories: 99 kcal  Protein: 4.75 g  Fat: 2.12 g Starches: 17.41 g

Ingredients

- *1\* 400g firm tofu, diced*
- *2 green onion, cut and corner to corner cut 1 10,000 foot stew, finely cleaved*
- *10g dried wakame 1L vegetable stock*
- *200g shiitake mushrooms, cut 120g miso paste*

Directions

a. Drench the wakame in tepid water for 10-15 minutes before depleting.

b. In a medium-sized pot include the vegetable stock and bring to the boil. Hurl in the mushrooms and stew for 2-3 minutes.

c. Blend miso paste with 3-4 tbsp of vegetable stock from the pan, until the miso is altogether broken up. Empty the miso-stock go into the container and include the tofu, wakame, green onions, and stew, at that point serve right away.

## 29. Mushroom and Tofu Scramble

Nutrition: Calories: 333 kcal Protein: 20.49 g Fat: 22.89 g Sugars: 18.83 g

Ingredients

- 50g mushrooms, daintily cut 5g parsley, finely cleaved
- 100g tofu, additional firm 1 tsp ground turmeric
- 1 tsp gentle curry powder 20g kale, generally cleaved 1 tsp additional virgin olive oil 20g red onion, daintily cut

Directions

a. Place 2 sheets of kitchen towel under and on the tofu, at that point rest an impressive weight, for example, pan onto the tofu, to guarantee it depletes off the fluid.

b. Join the curry powder, turmeric and 1-2 tsp of water to frame a paste. Utilizing a liner cook kale for 3-4 minutes.

c. In a pan, warm oil over medium warmth. Include the chili, mushrooms, and onion, cooking for a few minutes or until brown and delicate.

d. Break the tofu in too little pieces and hurl in the pan. Coat with the flavor paste and mix, guaranteeing everything turns out to be equally covered. Concoct for to 5 minutes, or until the tofu has cooked at that point include the kale and fry for 2 additional minutes. Embellishment with parsley before serving.

## 30.Buckwheat Pasta Salad

Nourishment: Calories: 440 kcal  Protein: 6.82 g  Fat: 39.33 g
Starches: 22.48 g

Ingredients
- 50g buckwheat pasta huge bunch of rocket
- 10 olives
- 1 tbsp additional virgin olive oil 20g pine nuts
- a little bunch of basil leaves
- 8 cherry tomatoes, split 1/2 avocado, diced

Directions

Join all the ingredients. Try not to incorporate the pine nuts. Orchestrate on a plate. Dissipate the pine nuts over the top.

# CONCLUSION

Of the a huge number of individuals who will follow popularized diets this year, under 1 percent will accomplish lasting weight loss. Not just do they neglect to have any kind of effect in the battle of the bulge, however they don't do anything to control the tsunami of interminable disease that has overwhelmed present day society.

We may live longer, but we are not living a healthy life. Stunningly, through the span of an insignificant ten years, the amount of time we spend in ill health has multiplied from 20% to 40%. It implies we currently spend 32 years of our lives in poor health. Simply take a look at the details. At this moment, one out of ten has diabetes and another three are close to getting it. Two out of each five individuals will be diagnosed with cancer at some phase in their lives. If you see three women beyond fifty one years old, one of them will have an osteoporotic crack. What's more, in the average time it takes you to peruse a single page of this book, a new case of Alzheimer's will build up and somebody will die of heart disease or coronary illness—and that is in the United States alone.

Consequently, "dieting" has never been our thing. That is, until we found Sirtfoods, a progressive new—and simple—approach to eat your way to weight reduction and stunning wellbeing.

The Sirtfood Diet book was first distributed in the U.K. in 2016. But, the United States release of the book has sparked more interest about the arrangement. The diet started getting publicity when Adele debuted her slimmer figure at the Billboard Music Awards last May. Her trainer, Pete Geracimo, is a colossal fanatic of the diet and says the singer shed thirty pounds from following a Sirt food diet. (Here, Adele gets genuine about getting healthy.)

As indicated by the book, this plan can assist you with burning fat and boost your vitality, preparing your body for long haul weight reduction achievement and a more healthy, disease-free life. All that while drinking red wine. Sounds like practically the ideal diet, isn't that so? All things considered, before you burn through your funds stocking up on sirtuins-filled fixings, know the pros and cons.